IT IS AIRBORNE

A Guide to Protecting You and Your Family from Airborne Diseases

ANTON WANG, PHARM.D., M.S.

Copyright © 2024 Anton Wang. All rights reserved.

No part of this publication may be reproduced, distributed, or transmitted in any form or by any means, including photocopying, recording, or other electronic or mechanical methods, without direct written permission from the author or publisher.

The information contained in this book is for informational purposes only. Under no circumstances will any blame or legal responsibility be held against the author or publisher. The author and publisher are not liable for any damages, reparation, or monetary loss arising out of or in connection with the use of this book. As always, you are responsible for your own choices, actions, and results.

ISBN-13: 9798321177259

First Edition

Medical Disclaimer and Liability Statement

THIS BOOK IS BASED ON THE AUTHOR'S PERSONAL THOUGHTS, RESEARCH, AND EXPERIENCES ONLY AND SHOULD NOT BE USED TO TAKE THE PLACE OF A MEDICAL PROFESSIONAL'S OPINION.

The author of this book has made every effort to provide accurate and up-to-date information. However, the author cannot guarantee that the information in this book is completely accurate or free from errors. The author is not liable for any damages or injuries that may result from the use of the information in this book, including, but not limited to, errors, omissions, or inaccuracies.

The reader is responsible for using their own judgment and discretion when using the information in this book. The reader should consult with a qualified medical professional before making any changes to their health care regimen.

The author of this book does not endorse any particular product or service. The author is not affiliated with any of the companies or organizations mentioned in this book.

The author of this book reserves the right to make changes to this book at any time. The reader is responsible for obtaining the most recent version of this book before using it.

By reading this book, the reader agrees to hold the author harmless from any liability for any damages or injuries that may result from the use of the information in this book.

CONTENTS

PREFACE..6

ACKNOWLEDGMENTS...9

INTRODUCTION..11

PART I: DEMYSTIFYING THE MISINFORMATION OF COVID-19

CHAPTER 1: Misinformation on the Characteristics of COVID-19......19
CHAPTER 2: The COVID-19 Pandemic and the Media's Role..........39

PART II: UNDERSTANDING COVID-19 AND LONG COVID

CHAPTER 3: Overview of COVID-19...51
CHAPTER 4: Long COVID: More Than Just a Cough....................65

PART III: PROTECTING YOURSELF, YOUR LOVED ONES, AND YOUR COMMUNITY

CHAPTER 5: Masking: Beyond Individual Choice..........................83
CHAPTER 6: Clean Air..97

EPILOGUE: A Ripple of Hope...111

NOTES..115

PREFACE

The COVID-19 pandemic has been a global crisis shrouded in misinformation. This book cuts through the noise to provide clear, evidence-based information about the virus and its effects. Leveraging my background in science, I will debunk common misinformation and equip you with the scientific understanding to make informed decisions for yourself and your loved ones.

I wrote this book for three main reasons:

- **To be a source of truth**: This book aims to be your trusted resource for understanding the complexities of COVID-19. It equips you with the knowledge to make informed decisions and ultimately reduce the risk of infection.
- **To validate your concerns**: You're not alone in questioning misinformation and unsubstantiated claims. This book aims to address those concerns with clear scientific evidence.
- **To empower you for action**: Armed with knowledge, we can navigate this pandemic together. You'll learn how to protect yourself, understand the long-term impacts of COVID-19, and even become a force for positive change.

This book is designed to empower everyone, regardless of scientific background, with a clear understanding of COVID-19.

- Part 1 tackles misinformation surrounding COVID-19, and explores how media coverage has impacted public perception.
- Part 2 provides an overview of COVID-19, and discusses its potential long-term effects.

- Part 3 explores practical strategies to safeguard yourself and your family from COVID-19. This includes the importance of high-quality masks, ventilation, and filtration.

This book isn't about politics, it's about education and action. Be prepared to encounter new information that may challenge your current understanding. After all, that's how we learn and grow. Ultimately, this book empowers you to make informed decisions to protect yourself and your loved ones, not just from COVID-19, but also from other airborne illnesses. Together, we can navigate this pandemic on a path of hope.

Sincerely,

Anton Wang, PharmD, MS

ACKNOWLEDGMENTS

I am incredibly grateful to my family for their unwavering love and support. Their patience, guidance, and inspiration have been instrumental in shaping who I am today.

I thank Dawn Jungemann and Linda R. S. Shepherd for reviewing this book, and extend my deepest thanks to Linda in particular for her unwavering support and encouragement throughout the writing journey. Her kind words were a source of strength, particularly during moments of doubt. This book is dedicated to the people and children of the world, in the hope that it may inspire positive change.

Finally, I want to acknowledge the profound influence of my past teachers and mentors. They instilled in me the importance of perseverance and always doing the right thing, principles that continue to guide me. I am also deeply inspired by the ongoing activism of countless individuals who fight for a better future. Especially during these challenging times, their spirit gives me hope.

INTRODUCTION

SARS-CoV-2 and COVID-19 are often used interchangeably, but they are not the same thing. **SARS-CoV-2 stands for Severe Acute Respiratory Syndrome Coronavirus 2**. It is the virus that causes **COVID-19, which stands for Coronavirus Disease 2019**. COVID-19 is the disease that SARS-CoV-2 can cause. In this book, I will use the terms SARS-CoV-2 and COVID-19 interchangeably, unless it is important to make a distinction between the two. I will avoid jargon and technical language whenever possible, and I will provide examples and analogies to help people understand the concepts at a deeper level.

To understand SARS-CoV-2, we need to learn about the history of SARS-CoV-1.

What is SARS-CoV-1?

SARS-CoV-1, also known as Severe Acute Respiratory Syndrome Coronavirus 1, is a respiratory virus that causes a respiratory illness called severe acute respiratory syndrome (SARS). The name coronavirus was inspired by the crown-shaped appearance of the spike glycoproteins on the virion surface when viewed under the electron microscope. SARS-CoV-1 was first identified in November 2002 in Foshan City, Guangdong Province, China. It spread rapidly worldwide but mostly to Asian countries before it was contained in July 2003. SARS-CoV-1 had an approximate case fatality rate of about 10%.[1] This means that about 1 in 10 people who were infected with SARS-CoV-1 died from the disease.

The World Health Organization (WHO) named the virus SARS-CoV-1 because it can cause a serious respiratory illness that can quickly get worse. Symptoms of SARS-CoV-1 can include fever, chills, shaking, cough, and dizziness. In some cases, SARS-CoV-1 can also cause lung inflammation and damage, which can lead to acute respiratory distress syndrome.[2]

Other symptoms of SARS-CoV-1 can include moderate lymphopenia (low levels of white blood cells), thrombocytopenia (low levels of platelets), a prolonged activated partial thromboplastin time (a blood test that measures how long it takes for blood to clot), elevated lactate dehydrogenase and creatine kinase levels (enzymes that are released when muscles are damaged), and elevated alanine aminotransferase levels (an enzyme that is released when the liver is damaged).[2] Fortunately, SARS-CoV-1 was a relatively short-lived outbreak. It lasted for about six months before it was contained.

Origin of SARS-CoV-1

Scientists believe that SARS-CoV-1 may have originated in bats. Bats are known to carry coronaviruses, and it is possible that SARS-CoV-1 evolved in bats and then jumped to humans. It is believed that the virus jumped from bats to civets, a small mammal that is sold as food in certain regions of China. From civets, the virus spread to humans.[3]

How is SARS-CoV-1 transmitted?

SARS-CoV-1 is transmitted via airborne particles produced when an infected person coughs or sneezes. It can also spread through contact with contaminated surfaces. The mean incubation period was about 6 days, ranging from 2 to 10 days.[1] The relatively prolonged incubation period allowed asymptomatic air travelers to spread the disease globally.

How was SARS-CoV-1 contained?

Nosocomial infection, also known as hospital-acquired infection or healthcare-associated infection, is an infection that is acquired in a hospital or other healthcare facility. It is a major problem in healthcare settings, and can be caused by a variety of factors, including contaminated air, the presence of other patients with infections, and the improper use of personal protective equipment (PPE).

Additionally, the SARS-CoV-1 outbreak was particularly challenging to control because it was a new virus and there was no specific treatment or vaccine available at the time. However, the public health measures implemented for SARS-CoV-1 were effective in slowing the spread of the virus and preventing a wider outbreak. The SARS-CoV-1 outbreak was contained through effective control of nosocomial infection and control of transmission in the community.

Effective control of nosocomial infection. This involved early detection of disease, strict isolation of patients, and the practice of airborne and contact precautions. It also required healthcare workers to comply with the use of PPE.

- **Early detection of disease.** This involved screening patients for symptoms of SARS-CoV-1 infection, such as fever, cough, and shortness of breath.
- **Strict isolation of patients.** Patients with SARS-CoV-1 infection were isolated in negative pressure rooms to prevent the spread of the virus to other patients and healthcare workers.

- **Airborne and contact precautions**. Healthcare workers caring for patients with SARS-CoV-1 infection were required to wear PPE, including gowns, gloves, masks, and eye protection. They also had to follow strict airborne and contact precautions, such as washing their hands frequently and avoiding contact with the patient's respiratory secretions.
- **Compliance with the use of PPE**. Healthcare workers need to use PPE correctly and consistently to protect themselves and their patients from infection.

Control of transmission in the community. This included tracing and quarantine of people who may have been exposed to the virus, as well as population adherence to widespread mask wearing and increased hygiene measures.

- **Tracing and quarantine of people who may have been exposed to the virus**. This involved identifying people who had close contact with a patient with SARS-CoV-1 infection and requiring them to quarantine.
- **Population adherence to widespread mask wearing**. Mask wearing is an effective way to reduce the spread of respiratory viruses, such as SARS-CoV-1.
- **Increased hygiene measures**. This involved washing hands frequently, avoiding touching your face, and covering your mouth and nose when you cough or sneeze.

The SARS-CoV-1 outbreak was a major public health challenge, but it was ultimately contained through a combination of effective public health measures. SARS-CoV-1 taught us a lot about coronaviruses and how to contain them. These measures were successful in slowing the spread of the virus and preventing a global pandemic. These measures can also be used to contain future outbreaks of respiratory viruses. However, for SARS-CoV-2, these measures were not implemented in sync across the globe and there was a delay in recognizing that the virus was primarily transmitted airborne.

Genetic similarity of SARS-CoV-2 versus SARS-CoV-1

SARS-CoV-2, the virus responsible for COVID-19, shares approximately 79% genetic similarity with SARS-CoV-1, the virus behind the 2003 SARS outbreak. Both viruses possess compact genomes of roughly 30,000 base pairs, essentially blueprints for their construction. Notably, their spike proteins, crucial for cell entry, contain around 1200-1300 amino acids.[4] This shared protein target explains their common entry point into human cells, via angiotensin-converting enzyme 2 (ACE2) receptors on cell surfaces.[5]

ACE2 receptors serve as a widespread gateway for SARS-CoV-2 infection, dotting cells of the upper respiratory tract to the deepest recesses of the lungs. In the airways, they are on the epithelial cells of the trachea and reside within the delicate air sacs known as alveoli. ACE2 receptors extend beyond the lungs, as they can be found in the endothelial cells of blood vessels, immune cells like monocytes and macrophages, and even brain cells. ACE2 expression is far and wide, including kidneys and the mucosal lining of the intestines. This extensive distribution explains why SARS-CoV-2 can invade such diverse organs and tissues and cause a myriad of symptoms. Upon infiltrating these diverse cells, the virus matures and unleashes its progeny, ready to embark on a new infectious journey.[5]

Despite the genetic similarity to its cousin, SARS-CoV-1, SARS-CoV-2 is a novel virus that has increased transmissibility and persistence.[6,7] It stubbornly lingers in bodies and the environment, creating more chances for havoc. This enhanced transmissibility and persistence make achieving immunity elusive and underscore the need for continued vigilance. This, coupled with its tendency to genetically mutate rapidly to form new variants, makes achieving lasting herd immunity through natural infection improbable.[8]

SARS-CoV-2 presents unique threats with potentially serious consequences. We must remember that the pandemic is not over, even if some media headlines suggest otherwise. New research raises concerning possibilities of permanent damage to the brain and body, a risk we shouldn't downplay.

The question isn't "how to live with the virus" or "how to control the virus," but "how do we live safely and responsibly with this ongoing threat"? Should we simply abandon attempts to contain nosocomial infections and community transmission? Should we allow SARS-CoV-2 to run rampant, jeopardizing lifespans and quality of life? Does "living with the virus" mean accepting repeated illnesses and potential disabilities for everyone, especially our most vulnerable populations – the elderly, children, and those with pre-existing conditions?

The human race isn't doomed to decimation by ignorance. We have the solutions – effective control measures and clean air initiatives – but implementing them requires collective will. This book aims to inspire a societal shift, advocating for clean air in all settings and prompting a renewed commitment to responsible pandemic management.

PART I

DEMYSTIFYING THE MISINFORMATION OF COVID-19

CHAPTER 1

Misinformation on the Characteristics of COVID-19

~~~
*"The repeated lie becomes the accepted reality."*
*- Aldous Huxley*
~~~

Do you have an open mind? If so, I encourage you to read this entire book. I understand that you may disagree with some of the information presented, and that is perfectly fine. The goal of this book is to provide you with information so that you can make informed decisions about COVID-19.

The COVID-19 pandemic has been a time of great misinformation. Since the beginning of the pandemic, people have been bombarded with false information about the virus, its origins, and how to prevent it. This misinformation has been spread through social media, news outlets, and even by some government officials.

The power of suggestion is real. When we are repeatedly exposed to the same information, our brains start to believe it. This is why it is so important to be critical of the information we consume. We need to be able to think for ourselves and evaluate the information we are given.

I encourage you to read this chapter with an open mind. I want you to be able to make informed decisions about COVID-19. I want you to be able to protect yourself and your loved ones.

In the next few chapters, we will examine the common misinformation surrounding COVID-19. We will focus on the key concepts, rather than trying to counter every piece of misinformation out there. The goal is to provide you with the source of truth and equip you with the ability to consider things from as many angles as possible to decipher whether a piece of information is a lie or truth. I hope that this book will help you to stay informed about COVID-19 and to make informed decisions about your health.

Below is a list of the misinformation that will be covered in this chapter:

Misinformation on the characteristics of COVID-19

- Misinformation: COVID-19 is a hoax.
- Misinformation: COVID-19 is over.
- Misinformation: COVID-19 is not airborne.
- Misinformation: COVID-19 is airborne, but that's not the main way it spreads.
- Misinformation: Viruses naturally evolve to become less deadly.
- Misinformation: COVID-19 is just like the flu and it is not as deadly as the flu.
- Misinformation: You can't get COVID-19 twice.
- Misinformation: Reinfections are rare.
- Misinformation: Breakthrough infections after vaccination are rare.
- Misinformation: Reinfections and breakthrough infections happen, but they're mild.

- Misinformation: Children don't get COVID-19 and they can't spread it.
- Misinformation: Once enough people have been exposed to COVID-19, herd immunity will end the pandemic.

Do any of the above statements sound familiar? Have you heard them from somewhere? We are living in a misinformation age, where bad actors are spreading misinformation to give the masses a false sense of security and illusion to prevent panic. COVID-19 is not over, despite what other people tell you or what you read. Let's take a deep dive into these misinformed statements.

Misinformation: COVID-19 is a hoax.

The harmful assertion that COVID-19 is fake has circulated online and in some communities, putting lives at risk. This misconception has no basis in science and can lead to ignoring safety measures. In reality, COVID-19 is a real and deadly virus responsible for over 7 million reported deaths worldwide by the end of 2023, according to the World Health Organization (WHO) COVID-19 dashboard.[1] The true number is likely even higher due to reporting discrepancies. Beyond the tragic death toll, millions more suffer from long-term health complications from the virus. Let's combat misinformation by relying on trusted sources and taking steps to protect ourselves and others. Don't let dangerous myths fuel the pandemic.

Misinformation: COVID-19 is over.

While many yearn for life pre-pandemic, the truth is that COVID-19 isn't done with us yet. The virus continues to circulate, infecting and claiming lives. Relaxed infection control measures in hospitals and communities could expose millions to potentially dangerous new variants.

Moreover, COVID-19's legacy isn't limited to the acute phase. As of October 2023, a staggering 5.3% of US adults, roughly 14 million people, grapple with long COVID.[2] This condition leaves lasting effects on multiple organs, potentially for years. This information is located on the CDC website. Search for "Guidance for Certifying Deaths Due to Coronavirus Disease" released February 27, 2023. A key paragraph states: "Emerging evidence suggests that SARS-CoV-2, the virus that causes COVID-19, can have lasting effects on nearly every organ and organ system of the body weeks, months, and potentially years after infection."[3]

COVID-19 is not just a short-term illness; it can be both acute and chronic. Misinformation, pandemic fatigue, and the desire for normalcy likely fuel the misconception that it's over. Remember, COVID-19 remains a serious threat, even for young and healthy individuals. It's crucial to remain informed, adopt preventive measures, and avoid spreading misinformation.

Misinformation: COVID-19 is not airborne.

COVID-19 is highly airborne, meaning it can spread easily through tiny respiratory droplets and aerosols released when an infected person breathes, talks, coughs, or sneezes. These particles can linger in the air for extended periods and travel much farther than the often-cited six feet, making social distancing and handwashing alone insufficient for controlling transmission.

Understanding airborne transmission is crucial for effective prevention. Good ventilation and mask-wearing become essential tools to curb the spread and protect individuals, especially in indoor settings. Dismissing the airborne nature of COVID-19 was a critical public health misstep that likely contributed to the virus's rapid spread. Just like influenza and RSV, SARS-CoV-2 thrives in the air.

Overwhelming scientific evidence confirms COVID-19's airborne transmission. Numerous studies have documented the presence of infectious virus particles in aerosols and their ability to travel long distances. One study performed in experimental laboratories suggests retained infectivity and virion integrity of COVID-19 for up to 16 hours in respirable-sized aerosols.[4]

In October 2023, 60 Minutes aired a segment highlighting the importance of indoor air quality in controlling COVID-19 and other airborne viruses like flu. Aerosol researchers emphasized the need to improve indoor air quality as a crucial prevention measure.

Here are some ways you could protect yourself and others:

- Wear a well-fitting mask, especially in indoor settings or crowded spaces. Masks significantly reduce the risk of inhaling airborne virus particles.
- Prioritize good ventilation. Open windows and doors whenever possible, and consider using air purifiers with HEPA filters in enclosed spaces.
- Stay informed and dispel misinformation. Share accurate information about COVID-19 transmission and prevention measures to help protect yourself and others.

Remember: Public health efforts over the past century have significantly improved air and water quality, but indoor air quality remains a critical concern. By recognizing the airborne nature of COVID-19 and taking appropriate precautions, we can better control its spread and protect ourselves and our communities.

Misinformation: COVID-19 is airborne, but that's not the main way it spreads.

Viral respiratory diseases, including influenza and SARS-CoV-2, can spread through close contact, short-range droplets, or long-range aerosols.[5]

- By contact: This involves touching a contaminated surface, like a doorknob, and then touching your eyes, nose, or mouth.
- By droplets: This happens when you breathe in tiny droplets released when an infected person coughs, sneezes, or talks. These droplets can land in your nose, mouth, or eyes.
- By aerosols: These are even tinier particles that can stay airborne for longer and travel further. You can inhale them into your upper or lower airways.

While some claim touching contaminated surfaces is the primary route for COVID-19 transmission, the truth is more nuanced. While contact can play a role, airborne transmission through respiratory droplets and aerosols remains the leading mode of transmission. A study investigates a superspreading event in March 2020, involving a choir practice in Skagit Valley, Washington, USA, where 53 of 61 unmasked attendees (87%) contracted COVID-19 despite taking precautions like physical distancing and hand hygiene. The poorly ventilated practice space allowed aerosols to linger, increasing the spread of COVID-19. The study concludes that aerosol inhalation was the primary mode of transmission. Additionally, the study highlights the importance of mask-wearing and proper ventilation in indoor settings to mitigate the spread of COVID-19.[6]

Understanding the Difference: Respiratory Droplets vs. Aerosols in Disease Transmission

- **Respiratory droplets**: Respiratory droplets are produced when a person breathes, coughs, sneezes, speaks, sings, or exercises. These droplets can contain viruses that cause infection.
- **Aerosols**: Aerosols are created when respiratory droplets evaporate. These aerosols can also contain viruses that cause infection.
- **Size**: Respiratory droplets are typically larger than aerosols, with a diameter of 5 micrometers or more. Aerosols, on the other hand, can be much smaller, with a diameter of less than 5 micrometers.
- **Distance traveled**: Respiratory droplets typically travel shorter distances than aerosols. Larger droplets can fall to the ground within seconds, while smaller droplets can stay suspended in the air for longer periods. Aerosols can travel long distances, depending on the environment.

It is important to note that these are just general guidelines. The size and distance traveled by respiratory droplets and aerosols can vary depending on several factors, such as the force of the person's exhalation, the humidity of the air, wind speed, wind direction, and the presence of other particles in the air.

It is also important to understand that while we encounter bacteria, fungi, and viruses daily, infection isn't simply a matter of exposure. It's a complex interplay between the highly infectious individual, the amount of viral particles they emit, the environmental factors like crowd density and ventilation, our body's robust immune system, and the dose and duration of inhalation. The denser the crowd, the higher the viral load, and the longer your exposure – the significantly higher your risk of infection. Understanding these factors empowers us to make informed choices, like wearing masks to protect ourselves from illness.

Misinformation: Viruses naturally evolve to become less deadly.

This is not always the case. Some viruses may evolve to become less deadly over time. This is because viruses that kill their hosts too quickly may not have a chance to spread to other hosts. However, other viruses, like HIV, can evolve to become more deadly over time. This is because viruses that can evade the immune system are more likely to survive and spread.

In the case of COVID-19, increasing evidence suggests concerning trends regarding the virus and its variants' ability to circumvent and damage the immune system. This raises concerns about potential increases in disease severity over time. The ongoing mutation of SARS-CoV-2, coupled with the rise of immune-evasive variants and the potential for repeated infections, raises serious concerns about the virus's long-term impact. Reinfections are a growing reality, posing health risks both in the acute and chronic phases. This repeated exposure, combined with the virus's ability to damage the immune system, raises the specter of cumulative harm to human health.[7]

Recent evidence suggests that COVID-19 is becoming more deadly as it evades and damages the immune system. Research shows SARS-CoV-2 can infect and damage T cells, crucial white blood cells for fighting infections.[8] T cells help to fight off infections by recognizing and attacking foreign invaders, such as viruses. SARS-CoV-2 infection may lead to:

- T-cell death: Weakening the body's immune response and increasing susceptibility to other infections.
- Lymphopenia: Reduced white blood cell count, further lowering infection-fighting capacity.

- Viral spread: Infected T cells may carry the virus throughout the body, potentially causing additional organ damage.

Damage to T cells can make it more difficult for the body to fight off infections. This can lead to more severe disease and a higher risk of death. Additionally, this can also lead to opportunistic infections to be more severe. While predicting future evolution is challenging, understanding these mechanisms highlights the potential seriousness of COVID-19's immune system evasion. Continued research and surveillance are crucial to assessing long-term implications and informing public health measures.

Misinformation: COVID-19 is just like the flu and it is not as deadly as the flu.

The initial symptoms of a disease do not define the disease. Don't be fooled by a mild start. Unlike the flu, COVID-19's impact can reach far beyond its initial symptoms, potentially causing lasting health problems even in those who feel fine at first. COVID-19 can initially present with symptoms similar to the flu, but it is a much more serious disease. New evidence shows that COVID-19 can damage the brain, vascular system, and immune system. This can lead to a range of long-term health problems, including long COVID, which is a condition that can cause fatigue, shortness of breath, and other symptoms for months or even years after infection.[9] Current treatments only help to alleviate the symptoms of long COVID, but there is no cure for long COVID.

Here are some of the key differences between COVID-19 and the flu[9-11]:

- COVID-19 is more contagious than the flu.

- COVID-19 can cause more severe illness than the flu. COVID-19 can cause a range of symptoms, including fever, cough, shortness of breath, fatigue, muscle aches, headache, sore throat, and loss of taste or smell. In some cases, COVID-19 can lead to dementia, stroke, heart attacks, pneumonia, acute respiratory distress syndrome, and death.
- COVID-19's reach extends beyond immediate illness, potentially causing lasting health issues even in mild cases. Some people who have been infected with COVID-19 have reported long-term health problems, including fatigue, shortness of breath, and difficulty thinking. These problems can last for weeks, months, or years after the initial illness.

While some COVID-19 symptoms can resemble the flu, like fever and cough, it's important to remember it's a different beast. Beyond the initial discomfort, COVID-19 can leave a long-term footprint on your health, even after a mild case. Think fatigue, brain fog, breathing difficulties, and more. It's like the flu with a hidden, potentially lingering impact.

Misinformation: You can't get COVID-19 twice.

It's a common misconception that getting COVID-19 once makes you immune forever. In reality, reinfection is possible, and even becoming infected multiple times. It is possible to get COVID-19 twice and even more, even if you have been previously infected or vaccinated. This is because the virus can mutate, and your body's immune system may not be able to recognize the new variant. There have been reports of people who have been infected with COVID-19 twice and even more. In some cases, subsequent reinfections may be more severe. Research evidence shows that reinfection further increases risks of death, hospitalization, and sequelae in multiple organ systems in the acute and chronic phases. Reducing the overall burden of death and disease due to SARS-CoV-2 will require strategies for reinfection prevention.

Why can this happen?

- Viral mutations: The SARS-CoV-2 virus, like many others, constantly evolves. These mutations can create new variants that your immune system, even if previously exposed or vaccinated, may not fully recognize.
- Waning immunity: Over time, the protection built up from a previous infection or vaccination can weaken. This allows the virus to potentially sneak past your defenses and reinfect you.

Growing evidence shows documented cases of individuals getting COVID-19 twice, three times, or even more.[7] Research suggests potential increases in risks like:

- Death: Studies indicate a higher risk of death after reinfection.
- Hospitalization: The need for hospitalization might be greater in subsequent infections.
- Organ damage: Long-term consequences like multiple organ system sequelae can occur in both the acute and post-acute phases after reinfection.

Misinformation: Reinfections are rare.

The idea that reinfections with COVID-19 are rare might seem logical, but reality paints a different picture. As the virus constantly evolves, reinfections are becoming increasingly common, especially with the emergence of new variants.

Why the Surge in Reinfections?

- **Rapid Evolution and Variants of Concern (VOCs)**: Unlike a static enemy, COVID-19 is a master of disguise. It mutates easily, creating almost infinite variant possibilities. The World Health Organization (WHO) closely monitors the virus, identifying specific VOCs with the potential to cause reinfections. Familiar names like Alpha, Beta, Gamma, Delta, and the recent Omicron (with its subvariants) all fall under this category.[12]
- **Immune Evasion and Damage**: For instance, the Omicron variant can skip acquired immunity from prior infection, hence increasing the risk of reinfection.[13] The immune system is designed to recognize viruses, but not all variants of a virus. Recall that COVID-19 is becoming more deadly as it evades and damages the immune system. Research shows SARS-CoV-2 can infect and damage T cells, crucial white blood cells for fighting infections.[8]

Reinfections make COVID-19 a challenging virus to fight. It is like a cat-and-mouse game, where the immune system is the cat and the virus is the mouse. The virus constantly mutates, trying to evade the immune system. The immune system constantly adapts, trying to recognize the new variants. The combination of COVID-19's rapid evolution and its ability to evade and damage the immune system over time raises serious concerns.

Remember, reinfections are a growing reality in the ever-changing landscape of COVID-19. By understanding the evolving enemy and implementing effective prevention measures, we can protect ourselves and others from the consequences of this persistent threat.

Misinformation: Breakthrough infections after vaccination are rare.

A breakthrough infection is a case where a person who has been "fully" vaccinated against a particular disease still contracts that disease. Technically, the term "fully" does not apply to SARS-CoV-2, since it is circulating widely and rapidly mutating. COVID-19 breakthrough infections in vaccinated individuals and reinfections in previously infected individuals have become increasingly common.[14]

Here are some of the common reasons for breakthrough infections:

- **Individual factors**: Some people's immune systems may not respond as well to vaccines as others. This can be due to factors like age, underlying health conditions, or medications that suppress the immune system.
- **Viral mutations**: Viruses can mutate over time, and new variants may emerge that can evade the immune response generated by a vaccine. This is what happened with the Omicron variant of the COVID-19 virus, for example.
- **Time since vaccination**: The protection provided by vaccines can wane over time, so someone who was fully vaccinated months or years ago may be more susceptible to a breakthrough infection than someone who was recently vaccinated.
- **Inadequate vaccine coverage**: If not enough people in a community are vaccinated, the virus can continue to circulate and there is a higher risk of breakthrough infections, even in people who are vaccinated.

Vaccines are like bulletproof vests. They can help protect you from getting seriously injured or killed, but they won't always stop a bullet from hitting you. The same is true for COVID-19 vaccines.

They can help protect you from getting seriously ill or dying from COVID-19, but they won't always stop you from getting infected. This is because vaccines work by training your body's immune system to recognize the virus that causes COVID-19. When you get vaccinated, your body produces antibodies that can fight off the virus if you are exposed to it. However, the virus that causes COVID-19 is constantly mutating. This means that the antibodies your body produces may not be effective against new virus variants.

While vaccines are effective in reducing the severity of COVID-19 and protecting vulnerable populations, no vaccine is 100% perfect. Viral evolution, the emergence of new variants, and individual immune response variations will require a multi-pronged approach beyond vaccination alone. This includes public health interventions like mask-wearing, clean indoor air, and improved ventilation to reduce airborne transmission.

Misinformation: Reinfections and breakthrough infections happen, but they're mild.

The statement that reinfections and breakthrough infections happen, but they're mild is a dangerous myth. Reinfections and breakthrough infections can happen to anyone, regardless of vaccination status. Even if a reinfection or breakthrough infection is "mild", it can still lead to long-term health problems, such as long COVID. Beyond the initial illness, COVID-19 can leave a significant legacy. Long COVID, affecting at least 10% of cases, encompasses over 200 symptoms across various organ systems, potentially leading to lasting and debilitating health challenges.[15]

Diseases such as hepatitis C, HIV, and Lyme disease, can initially present with "mild" symptoms similar to the flu. However, these diseases can progress to cause serious lifelong health problems, such as liver damage, AIDS, and neurological disorders. Imagine surviving COVID-19, only to be haunted by its shadow months later. That's Long COVID, a debilitating illness affecting at least 10% of those infected. With over 200 symptoms ranging from fatigue to organ damage, it's a complex condition that shouldn't be treated lightly.

Additionally, asymptomatic COVID-19 cases can contribute to the spread of the virus.[16] While their infectivity may vary compared to symptomatic cases, the ability to transmit the virus without experiencing symptoms highlights the importance of precautions including masking to protect others, even if you feel well.

Misinformation: Children don't get COVID-19 and they can't spread it

It's important to set the record straight: Children can and do get COVID-19, and they can also spread the virus to others. This misinformation puts children at risk, as it can lead to delayed diagnosis, inadequate care, and potential long-term health consequences.

Millions of children in the U.S. have experienced long COVID after contracting the virus. This means they can have lingering symptoms for months, even after recovering from the initial illness.[17] These symptoms vary but can include:

- Persistent fatigue
- Cough that doesn't go away
- Headaches
- Loss of taste or smell
- Dizziness or lightheadedness
- Worsening of existing health conditions

Long COVID can also lead to new conditions in children, including:

- Postural orthostatic tachycardia syndrome (POTS): Feeling faint upon standing
- Chronic fatigue syndrome: Extreme tiredness and muscle aches
- Autoimmune conditions: Problems with the immune system attacking healthy tissues
- Multisystem inflammatory syndrome (MIS-C): Severe inflammation throughout the body

It's crucial to acknowledge that long COVID can also affect children's mental and emotional well-being, potentially leading to increased anxiety or depression. If you suspect your child might have long COVID, don't hesitate to talk to their doctor. They can help diagnose the problem, manage symptoms, and offer support during this challenging time.

There are some things that parents can do to protect their children from the serious health risks of COVID-19. These include:

- Get their children vaccinated against COVID-19.
- Make sure their children wear well-fitted, high-quality masks in public.
- Make sure indoor air is well-ventilated and has a HEPA air purifier running to reduce airborne viral load.
- Avoid crowded indoor spaces.
- Get their children tested for COVID-19 if they have symptoms.

By dispelling misinformation and taking preventive measures, we can create a safer and healthier environment for all children.

Misinformation: Once enough people have been exposed to COVID-19, herd immunity will end the pandemic.

The idea that once enough people have been exposed to COVID-19, herd immunity will end the pandemic is a dangerous myth. Herd immunity is a theoretical concept that refers to the point at which enough people in a population are immune to a disease that it can no longer spread easily. However, it is theoretically impossible to achieve herd immunity for a virus like COVID-19. The virus is constantly mutating, and the rate of mutation increases with an increasing number of infected human hosts. Additionally, the virus can evade and damage the body's immune system, making it difficult for the body to develop lasting immunity.

Herd immunity alone cannot completely end the pandemic.[18] Achieving herd immunity through natural exposure or a vaccine-only strategy is risky and unreliable for the following reasons:

- It can lead to high numbers of serious illnesses, hospitalizations, and deaths, especially among vulnerable populations.
- The long-term effects of COVID-19 are still being understood, and relying on widespread infection or a vaccine-only strategy isn't a responsible approach.
- Viral mutations and the emergence of new variants can undermine herd immunity achieved through past infections or vaccinations.
- Reinfections are increasingly common, complicating herd immunity calculations.

Effective control measures and clean air initiatives are necessary for responsible pandemic management.

Seeds of Change

Welcome to the end of this chapter! You've tackled some tough topics about COVID-19 misinformation, uncovering the truth about viral mutation, herd immunity myths, and more. Take a breather before diving into the next chapter, letting your new knowledge settle in. You've armed yourself with powerful knowledge to fight misinformation and educate others.

As you journey through this book, stay curious and challenge your assumptions. Your open mind is the key to continued learning and making a difference.

Some key highlights of this chapter:

1. COVID-19 is a real and highly contagious disease caused by the SARS-CoV-2 virus. Millions of people worldwide have been infected, and the virus has caused millions of deaths. These numbers continue to increase.
2. COVID-19 remains a serious threat, even for young and healthy individuals.
3. COVID-19 is not just a short-term illness; it can be both acute and chronic.
4. COVID-19 is primarily airborne, spreading through respiratory droplets and aerosols released when an infected person exhales, coughs, sneezes, talks, or sings.
5. While touching contaminated surfaces remains a risk factor, COVID-19 airborne transmission is the major mode of spread. Mask-wearing remains a crucial preventative measure.
6. COVID-19 has become more deadly, with new variants emerging that are more transmissible and sometimes more virulent. Recent evidence suggests that COVID-19 is

becoming more deadly as it evades and damages the immune system.
7. While COVID-19 shares some symptoms with the flu, it is significantly more contagious and poses a higher risk of severe illness, hospitalization, and death, especially for vulnerable populations. Long-term health complications like long COVID are also a major concern.
8. Reinfections with COVID-19 are possible, even for previously infected individuals or vaccinated people. Even if a reinfection or breakthrough infection is "mild", it can still lead to long-term health problems, such as long COVID.
9. Asymptomatic COVID-19 cases can contribute to the spread of the virus.
10. The frequency of COVID-19 reinfections is increasing with the emergence of new variants that can evade immunity from previous infections or vaccinations.
11. Long COVID, affecting at least 10% of cases, encompasses over 200 symptoms across various organ systems, potentially leading to lasting and debilitating health challenges.
12. Children can and do get COVID-19, and they can also spread the virus to others. Millions of children in the U.S. have experienced long COVID after contracting the virus.
13. Achieving herd immunity through natural exposure is risky and unreliable. It can lead to high morbidity and mortality, especially among vulnerable populations. Effective control measures and clean air initiatives are necessary for responsible pandemic management.

CHAPTER 2

The COVID-19 Pandemic and the Media's Role

~~~
*"All media exist to invest our lives with artificial perceptions and arbitrary values." - Marshall McLuhan*
~~~

Living in a cloud of misinformation: The COVID-19 pandemic unleashed a torrent of misinformation, churning through social media, news outlets, and even official channels. From the virus's origins to prevention methods, false narratives proliferated, leaving many confused and vulnerable. This is particularly concerning because once misinformation takes root, it can be incredibly difficult to dislodge and replace with accurate information. After all, altering deeply ingrained perceptions and values is no easy feat.

The media's powerful influence: Mass media is a powerful sculptor of our perceptions and values. Constant exposure to advertising, for instance, can subtly condition us to equate happiness with material possessions. Through news coverage, entertainment, and advertising, the media bombards us with a steady stream of information and interpretations that shape our understanding of events, people, and even ourselves.

Cultivating critical thinking: Given the media's undeniable influence, cultivating critical thinking skills is paramount. We must approach information with skepticism, acknowledging how our own biases and assumptions color our worldview. This necessitates questioning media narratives and perspectives, actively seeking diverse sources, and considering alternative viewpoints.

Examining the media's role in the pandemic: This chapter delves into the media's role during the COVID-19 pandemic, exploring potential reasons behind news blackouts and misinformation campaigns. By understanding how our perceptions are shaped, we gain the power to influence our behaviors and potentially even the world around us.

Should you trust the media?

The media plays an important role in our society. It informs us about current events, helps us to understand the world around us, and holds those in power accountable. However, there has been a growing distrust of the media in recent years. Some people believe that the media is biased and that they cannot be trusted to provide accurate information.

There are some reasons why people might distrust the media. One reason is that the media is often owned by large corporations. These corporations have a vested interest in promoting certain viewpoints, and they may use their media outlets to do so. For example, a corporation that owns a news network might be more likely to report stories that are favorable to its business interests.

Another reason people might distrust the media is that the media is often funded by advertising. Advertisers want to reach a large audience, and they are willing to pay media outlets to promote their products or services. This can create a conflict of interest, as media outlets may be more likely to report stories that are favorable to their advertisers.

There are several things that people can do to make informed decisions about the information that they consume. First, people should be aware of the biases of the media outlets that they consume. Second, people should be critical of the information that they read and watch. They should ask themselves who is behind the information and what their motives might be. Third, people should get their news from a variety of sources. This will help to ensure that they are getting a balanced view of the news.

Who owns the media in the US?

The media in the United States is owned by a small number of large corporations. These corporations control the vast majority of the news outlets, television stations, and radio stations in the country. This gives them a significant amount of power to shape the public's understanding of the world. This concentration of ownership has led to concerns about the media's ability to provide independent and unbiased reporting.

The concentration of ownership in the media has several implications. First, it can lead to a lack of diversity in the news. When a small number of companies control most of the media, they are likely to promote the same viewpoints. This can make it difficult for people to get a balanced view of the news.

Second, the concentration of ownership can lead to a lack of accountability. When a small number of companies control the majority of the media, they are less likely to be held accountable for their reporting. This can make it easier for them to spread misinformation or to promote their self-seeking interests.

The concentration of ownership in the media is a serious problem. It undermines the public's ability to get accurate and unbiased information. It is important to be aware of this problem and to take steps to get your news from a variety of sources.

Why the media blacked out COVID news and misinformed the public

The COVID-19 pandemic has been a major news story for the past few years. However, there has been a noticeable decline in the amount of coverage that the pandemic receives. This decline in coverage has coincided with some public health experts warning that the pandemic is not over and that we are still at risk of a new surge in cases.

There are several possible explanations for why the media has blacked out COVID news. One possibility is that the media is simply tired of covering the pandemic. After a few years of constant coverage, the pandemic may have become old news for many people. Another possibility is that the media is under pressure from advertisers to focus on more positive stories. Advertisers are less likely to want to be associated with negative stories about the pandemic, and the media may be reluctant to lose their advertising revenue.

Whatever the reason, the decline in COVID news coverage is a problem. Without adequate coverage, the public is less likely to be aware of the risks of the pandemic and less likely to take steps to protect themselves. This could lead to a new surge in cases and deaths.

In addition to blacking out COVID news, the media has also been guilty of spreading misinformation about the pandemic. For example, some media outlets have downplayed the severity of the virus, claiming that it is no worse than the common cold. Others have promoted unproven treatments for the virus, such as hydroxychloroquine. This misinformation can be dangerous, as it can lead people to make decisions that put their health at risk.

The media has a responsibility to inform the public about the COVID-19 pandemic. However, by blacking out news and spreading misinformation, the media is failing to meet this responsibility. This is a serious problem that could have devastating consequences for society as a whole.

What can be done to address the media's manipulation?

Several things can be done to address the problem of the media blacking out COVID news and spreading misinformation. One thing that can be done is to hold the media accountable. This can be done by writing letters to the editor, calling into talk shows, and signing petitions. It is also important to support independent media outlets providing accurate and unbiased reporting on the pandemic.

Another thing that can be done is to educate the public about the importance of getting their news from reliable sources. People should be aware of the biases of the media outlets they consume and be critical of the information they read and watch. They should also be aware of the dangers of misinformation and should be careful about sharing information that they are not sure is true.

The media's illusory lens: masks off, pandemic on

A glimpse at media coverage could lull viewers into a false sense of normalcy. Interviewers and interviewees mingle, masks discarded, and the pandemic seems a distant memory. Yet, this carefully curated image obscures the harsh reality playing out just beyond the frame. The World Economic Forum (WEF) in Davos, with its strict health protocols, serves as one example of this discrepancy. While participants attending the WEF took significant precautions and held interviews without masks, the pandemic continues to pose serious challenges for people worldwide.

But beyond Davos, the media's role in amplifying this disparity deserves scrutiny. By presenting a sanitized version of reality, with masks cast aside and life seemingly back to normal, it peddles an artificial perception. This narrative can harm working people by downplaying the pandemic's ongoing threat and placing undue responsibility on individuals. Downplaying the virus obscures the potential consequences of workplace exposure, and sickness becomes a "personal responsibility."

The illusion of normalcy must be shattered. We must recognize the media's role in shaping perceptions and demand truthful narratives that acknowledge the pandemic's reality. We need the media to acknowledge both the progress made and the ongoing need for vigilance. This will help ensure responsible communication that promotes public health and fosters a more accurate understanding of the current situation.

Long COVID: A growing threat to our health and future

Long COVID, a serious and potentially life-altering condition, can impact any organ system and can cause potentially devastating lifelong consequences. With each COVID-19 infection, the risk of developing long COVID increases, raising concerns about individual and societal well-being. Each reinfection compounds the risk of developing long COVID. This invisible roulette threatens not only individuals but also their loved ones' ability to care for them and each other.

The impact of long COVID on individuals and families is unsettling. Imagine the financial and emotional burden of disability from long COVID. The potential domino effect of cascading disabilities raises serious concerns. Consider these questions:

- Who will care and provide for you if long COVID disables you?
- How will you care and provide for loved ones (parents, spouses, children) affected by long COVID?
- Why are we seemingly accepting long COVID as inevitable?

Each infection and reinfection of COVID-19 can have costly life and health insurance implications. It's no secret that insurers inquire about COVID-19 history. Their actuarial data reveals the increased risk of long COVID with each infection, translating to higher liability for them. This could lead to denied coverage, higher premiums, and financial strain for individuals. Notably, while media coverage often skips these details, the American Academy of Actuaries has acknowledged the anticipated rise in medical costs and premiums due to long COVID's diverse health impacts, including fatigue, organ damage, and increased mental health needs.[2]

It's time to say "enough is enough." Ignoring long COVID is no longer an option. We have the tools and we must protect ourselves and our loved ones from this virus and its potential long-term effects. We must advocate for increased awareness, research funding, and preventive measures to combat long COVID. Remember, long COVID often presents as fatigue, but it can also affect various organ systems and require mental health support. Let's urge action. We deserve to be protected from this virus and its long-term consequences. Let's say, "Enough is enough!" and protect our health and the well-being of our families.

Feeling powerless but hopeful in a leaky ship

Imagine shoveling coal into the Titanic's furnace, knowing full well it's gushing water and doomed to sink. That's the sinking feeling I get seeing the ongoing pandemic's mishandling. So, like tossing out life jackets to fellow passengers, I've dedicated myself to sharing what I know, hoping to better protect you and your loved ones.

Amazon built a high-tech headquarters in Arlington, Virginia, that monitors CO2 levels, pumping in fresh air the moment things get stuffy. They even filter out viruses, bacteria, and mold.[1] Imagine if such technology, not luxury yachts, became the norm! Democratizing clean indoor air for everyone, every workplace, school, gym, nursing home, restaurant – all equipped with high-grade filters and sound ventilation systems. It's not a pipe dream; it's a matter of prioritizing health and well-being over profit margins.

We can't control the storm, but we can build sturdy vessels. Let's work together to craft lifejackets of knowledge and lifeboats of accessible, clean air. We owe it to ourselves, our loved ones, and every passenger on this shared ship called Earth.

Remember, even the smallest actions can ripple outward. Sharing this message, demanding better air quality in your community, and supporting businesses prioritizing employee health are all strokes towards a healthier future. Together, we can weather this storm and build a world where clean air is a right, not a privilege.

Some key highlights of this chapter:

1. Mass media shapes our perceptions and values through news, entertainment, and advertising.

2. Cultivating critical thinking is crucial to navigate through biased information.
3. The decline in COVID-19 news coverage raises concerns about transparency and accountability.
4. Media outlets are often owned by large corporations with vested interests.
5. Blackouts and misinformation campaigns can have dire consequences for public health.
6. The media often presents a sanitized version of reality. This narrative can harm working people by downplaying the pandemic's ongoing threat and placing undue responsibility on individuals.
7. Life and health insurance companies may consider your COVID-19 history due to the increased risk of long COVID, potentially impacting coverage and cost.
8. The actuarial community anticipates rising insurance premiums and medical costs due to long COVID's wide-ranging health complications.
9. Democratizing clean air and prioritizing health over profit are essential goals.
10. Amazon's high-tech headquarters with advanced air filtration exemplifies unequal access to clean air.
11. Building a world where clean air is a right requires collective effort and systemic change.

PART II

UNDERSTANDING COVID-19 AND LONG COVID

CHAPTER 3

Overview of SARS-CoV-2

~~~
*"The first step in solving any problem is to understand it. And the only way to understand a problem is to understand its fundamentals. Once you understand the fundamentals, you can start to see the big picture. And once you see the big picture, you can start to come up with solutions."*
*- Richard Feynman*
~~~

Understanding the fundamentals: The human body is made up of trillions of cells, each of which is made up of billions of molecules. These molecules dynamically interact with one another in a complex web of interactions and reactions. We can better understand and prevent diseases when we unravel these complexities down to the fundamentals. It's like learning the alphabet before writing a sentence. Understanding the fundamentals of human biology and viruses is crucial before delving into the intricate interplay between them.

The master key of SARS-CoV-2: Think of the SARS-CoV-2 virus as a cunning lockpick, exploiting vulnerabilities in our cellular defenses. It has a "master key" for certain "locks" on our cells, called angiotensin-converting enzyme 2 (ACE2) receptors. By binding to these receptors, the virus gains entry and starts replicating, causing havoc within the cell. ACE2 receptors are involved in blood pressure regulation and they are ubiquitous throughout the body. This "master key" explains the diverse array of symptoms, from migraines to chest pain, experienced by individuals infected with the virus. By understanding how the virus uses its "master key" to manipulate these "locks" and the resulting cellular chaos, we gain invaluable insights into its behavior and potential weaknesses.

Seeing the big picture: This chapter delves into the hidden world of viruses, starting with the fundamental mechanisms of their life cycle. We'll then shift our focus to SARS-CoV-2, examining its unique ability to mutate and generate new variants. Finally, we'll critically assess current drug treatments and their limitations in combating this ever-evolving threat. This comprehensive understanding empowers us to see the bigger picture and develop effective strategies to protect ourselves and combat the virus on multiple fronts.

The general life cycle of a virus

Viruses are tiny organisms that can only replicate inside living cells. They are not alive in the traditional sense, but they can cause disease. When a virus enters a cell, it hijacks the cell's machinery to make copies of itself. This process can damage cells and lead to illness. The life cycle of a virus is the process by which it infects a cell, replicates, and then spreads to other cells.

The life cycle of a virus can be divided into the following stages[1]:

1. **Attachment**: The first step in the life cycle of a virus is attachment. The virus must attach to a specific receptor on the surface of a cell to infect it. The receptor is a protein that the virus recognizes and binds to. SARS-CoV-2 binds to the ACE2 receptors on the cell surface. ACE2 receptors' function is to modulate blood pressure and maintain blood

pressure homeostasis, which is why they are ubiquitous throughout the human body.

2. **Penetration**: Once the virus has attached to a cell, it penetrates the cell membrane. This can happen in several ways, including endocytosis, fusion, or injection. Endocytosis is a process by which the cell engulfs the virus particle. Fusion is a process by which the virus particle fuses with the cell membrane. Injection is a process by which the virus particle injects its genetic material into the cell. The COVID-19 virus enters a cell via fusion. The virus's spike protein binds to the ACE2 receptor on the surface of the cell. This binding triggers a conformational change in the spike protein, which exposes a fusion peptide. The fusion peptide then inserts itself into the cell membrane, causing the viral and cell membranes to fuse.

3. **Uncoating**: Once the virus has penetrated the cell, it uncoats. This means that the protein coat of the virus is removed, exposing the viral genome. The viral genome is made up of DNA or RNA. The COVID-19 virus is made up of RNA.

4. **Replication**: The viral genome is then replicated. This process is carried out by the cell's machinery, which has been hijacked by the virus. The COVID-19 virus is specifically a positive-sense, single-stranded RNA virus. This means that the RNA strand is read directly by the cell's ribosomes to produce proteins.

5. **Assembly**: Once the viral genome has been replicated, new virus particles are assembled. This process involves the production of new protein coats and the assembly of the viral genome into new virus particles. The new virus particles are made up of the same proteins and nucleic

acids as the original virus particle.

6. **Release**: The newly assembled virus particles are then released from the cell. This can happen in several ways, including lysis (bursting of the cell) or budding (the virus particles bud off from the cell membrane).

Once the virus particles have been released, they can then infect other cells and start the life cycle all over again. The life cycle of a virus can vary depending on the type of virus and the general steps are outlined above. The life cycle of a virus is a complex process that is essential for the virus to replicate and spread. Understanding the life cycle is crucial for developing prevention and treatment strategies. Masks can help prevent initial attachment and infection.

Here is a simple analogy that you can use to explain the life cycle of a virus to an 8-year-old child and to encourage your child to wear a mask for personal protection:

- Imagine a virus as a tiny burglar. The burglar wants to break into your house and steal your belongings. The burglar has a special key that can open any door in your house.
- Once inside the house, the burglar steals your belongings and can make copies of itself. The burglars then leave your house in ruin and start breaking into other houses in your neighborhood.
- The virus works similarly. Once the virus is inside your cells, it can start to replicate and spread throughout your body.
- Wearing a mask is like having a security gate to prevent the burglar from getting into your house in the first place.

Understanding SARS-CoV-2: Genetic blueprint, mutation, and recombination

The relentless emergence of SARS-CoV-2 variants poses a significant societal challenge. To effectively combat this threat, we must delve into the very core of the virus and understand its propensity for mutation.

Why does this matter? Reducing the number of human hosts infected with SARS-CoV-2 directly impacts its mutation rate. Each infection presents an opportunity for the virus to evolve, potentially creating new variants with unforeseen characteristics. The fewer hosts it infects, the less likely it is to mutate and potentially outpace existing vaccines and treatments. By lifting the hood on the virus and understanding its nature, we empower ourselves to create targeted strategies that minimize viral spread and reduce mutation opportunities.

The genetic blueprint of SARS-CoV-2:

- Viruses store their genetic information in either DNA or RNA. SARS-CoV-2, the virus responsible for COVID-19, utilizes positive-sense, single-stranded RNA. This RNA strand directly serves as a blueprint for protein production within infected cells.
- Compared to DNA viruses, RNA viruses like SARS-CoV-2 are simpler, lacking the protective protein shell (capsid) found in DNA viruses. Instead, they rely on a lipid envelope derived from the host cell.
- The SARS-CoV-2 RNA genome is relatively small, around 30,000 nucleotides, compared to DNA viruses like the herpes simplex virus with around 150,000 nucleotides.[2,3] Compared to DNA viruses, SARS-CoV-2's smaller genome size and single-stranded RNA nature make it more efficient in creating copies of itself.

Evolutionary mechanisms:

- **Mutation**: During replication, errors can occur in copying the RNA, leading to mutations. If these mutations affect protein-coding genes, they can alter the virus's structure and create new variants, potentially evading immune system recognition.
- **Recombination**: Recombination is a process that occurs when two different viruses of the same species combine their genetic material. When two different SARS-CoV-2 strains co-infect a cell, their genetic material can merge, generating hybrid viruses with unique combinations of genes from the two original viruses. This further fuels viral evolution.

Impact of evolution:

- The combined effect of mutation and recombination drives the emergence of new SARS-CoV-2 variants with diverse properties. These variants can exhibit increased transmissibility, virulence, and vaccine resistance, posing significant challenges to achieving herd immunity.
- The combined effect of mutation and recombination also complicates vaccine and treatment development, as strategies effective against one strain might not work against another. Hence, a vaccine-only strategy is not enough to contain the virus.[4]

While mutations are a key feature of viruses, it's theoretically impossible that SARS-CoV-2 will mutate itself to extinction. Imagine a virus making millions of copies within a cell. Even if a single mutation occurs, it has to compete with those "normal" copies to spread further. While the vast majority will remain functional, the mutated variant might offer an advantage or disadvantage in transmission or immune escape. Only if it provides a significant benefit will it outcompete the majority and become dominant. Therefore, while the virus will likely continue evolving, it's highly improbable that mutations will drive it to extinction. Instead, our focus should be on effective public health measures and clean air initiatives to limit transmission and reduce mutation opportunities.

Ribosome: a micro-machine for manufacturing proteins

A ribosome is a complex molecule found in all living cells, from bacteria to humans. It is responsible for protein synthesis by translating the genetic code into proteins. Ribosomes are made up of two subunits, a large subunit and a small subunit. The large subunit contains the enzymes that are needed to translate the genetic code, while the small subunit binds to the messenger RNA (mRNA) molecule that contains the genetic code. There can be as many as millions of ribosomes in a single human cell.

The ribosome reads the mRNA molecule one codon at a time. A codon is a sequence of three nucleotides that codes for a specific amino acid. The ribosome then uses the amino acids to build a protein. In simplicity, the protein is built in the ribosome in the following steps:

1. The ribosome binds to the mRNA molecule.
2. The ribosome reads the first codon on the mRNA molecule.
3. The ribosome uses the amino acids that are attached to the small subunit to match the codon on the mRNA molecule.
4. The ribosome adds the amino acid to the growing protein chain.
5. The ribosome moves to the next codon on the mRNA molecule.

6. Steps 3-5 are repeated until the entire protein has been built.
7. The ribosome releases the finished protein from the small subunit.

Ribosomes are essential for life and are composed of special proteins and nucleic acids. Without ribosomes, cells would not be able to produce proteins, and cells would not be able to function properly. Ribosomes are very efficient and can translate millions of codons per second. Ribosomes are found in the cytoplasm of cells and are also found in the endoplasmic reticulum. Understanding the basics of ribosomes helps us better understand how vaccines and viruses use cellular machinery for different purposes.

Understanding the difference: How SARS-CoV-2 and mRNA vaccines use ribosomes

While both SARS-CoV-2 and mRNA vaccines involve ribosomes, they use them in fundamentally different ways:

- SARS-CoV-2: The virus hijacks human ribosomes to produce complete copies of itself, enabling it to spread and infect new cells.
- mRNA vaccines: They deliver instructions (mRNA) that tell our ribosomes to create copies of just the spike protein, a component on the virus's surface. This triggers our immune system to build defenses against the actual virus, without causing infection.

The key takeaway lies in what's produced. SARS-CoV-2 replicates itself, while mRNA vaccines use ribosomes to train our immune system to recognize and fight the virus. Now that you have a basic understanding of the life cycle of a virus, SARS-CoV-2, and ribosomes, let's review some fundamentals of Paxlovid to understand why we cannot rely solely on drugs to reduce the transmission of SARS-CoV-2.

Paxlovid: A valuable tool in the fight against COVID-19, but not a magic bullet

Paxlovid is a combination drug that contains two active ingredients: nirmatrelvir and ritonavir. Each active ingredient serves a different purpose.

- Nirmatrelvir is a protease inhibitor that blocks the activity of a viral protein called Mpro. Mpro is essential for the replication of SARS-CoV-2. By blocking Mpro, nirmatrelvir prevents SARS-CoV-2 from replicating and spreading in the body.
- Ritonavir is a drug that is used to boost the concentration of nirmatrelvir in the blood. Ritonavir does not have any antiviral activity on its own, but it helps to prevent nirmatrelvir from being broken down by the body. This allows nirmatrelvir to stay in the body longer and more effectively prevent SARS-CoV-2 replication.[5]

Paxlovid offers hope in the fight against COVID-19. However, it's essential to understand its usefulness and limitations. Paxlovid is approved for adults and adolescents 12 years old and older with mild-to-moderate COVID-19 and high-risk factors for severe illness.[6] The eligibility criteria for Paxlovid include:

- Adults and adolescents (12 years of age and older and weighing at least 88 pounds)
- Has mild to moderate COVID-19
- Has one or more risk factors for progression to severe COVID-19
- Have symptoms for no more than 5 days since the start of

the illness

Paxlovid has shown promising results in clinical trials, reducing hospitalization and death risks.[7] However, it's crucial to remember:

- **Eligibility matters**: Paxlovid is not for everyone. Eligibility criteria include age, underlying health conditions, and symptom duration (within 5 days). Consult your healthcare provider to determine if it's right for you.
- **Not a cure**: While Paxlovid effectively combats the virus, it doesn't prevent long-term complications from a SARS-CoV-2 infection. Vaccination and public health measures remain crucial.
- **Side effects and drug interactions exist**: Paxlovid can cause side effects like taste changes and diarrhea, as well as unwanted drug interactions. Discuss potential risks and benefits with your healthcare provider.

Paxlovid plays a valuable role in managing COVID-19, but like any antiviral medication, its effectiveness can be affected by factors like viral mutations and persistence. It's essential to combine antiviral treatments with preventive measures like vaccination, masking, and ventilation to achieve optimal protection. By understanding Paxlovid's potential and limitations, we can make informed decisions about its role in our individual and collective fight against COVID-19.

COVID-19 rebound with Paxlovid: What you need to know

COVID-19 rebound refers to a phenomenon where people experience a return of symptoms or a positive test result after completing a course of Paxlovid. It's important to note that rebound is not caused by Paxlovid itself, but rather it reflects the natural course of the infection in some individuals.

Rebound symptoms are typically similar to the initial COVID-19 infection. Some common symptoms include:

- Cough
- Fatigue
- Fever
- Muscle aches
- Congestion

One study suggests that COVID-19 rebound might be more common than initially thought. Investigators found that approximately 1 in 5 participants who took Paxlovid experienced a rebound, and they also experienced prolonged viral shedding for an average of 14 days.[8]

Remember, even if you experience no symptoms, you can still be contagious during rebound. Anyone experiencing rebound symptoms or testing positive after finishing Paxlovid should:

- Get retested often and follow their healthcare provider's advice regarding re-testing.
- Isolate themselves and follow preventive measures to prevent transmission.
- Contact their healthcare provider for guidance and follow their recommendations, which may include isolating at home, monitoring symptoms, or seeking further medical care.

Despite the possibility of a rebound, Paxlovid remains a valuable tool in the fight against COVID-19, particularly for individuals at high risk of severe illness. If you're concerned about rebound or have any questions about Paxlovid, consult your healthcare provider for personalized advice based on your specific situation.

Empowering Parents: Protecting Children from COVID-19 Through Prevention

Paxlovid is currently unavailable for children under 12 years old or children 12 years and older who weigh less than 88 pounds. This means that these children would have to rely on their immunity for protection from COVID-19. This is a serious concern, as children are also at risk of developing long COVID and serious complications from COVID-19, including hospitalization and death. Growing concerns suggest potential long-term health effects from COVID-19, even in mild cases, making effective preventive measures even more crucial.[9]

There are some things that parents can do to protect their children from the serious health risks of COVID-19. These include:

- Get their children vaccinated against COVID-19.
- Make sure their children wear quality masks in public.
- Make sure indoor air is well-ventilated and has a HEPA air purifier running to reduce airborne viral load.
- Avoid crowded indoor spaces.
- Get their children tested for COVID-19 if they have symptoms.

By staying informed, taking precautions, and supporting clean air initiatives, we can work towards protecting children from COVID-19 and its potential long-term effects.

In summary, relying solely on vaccines, medications, and natural immunity to stop the COVID-19 pandemic is insufficient. Viral mutations and waning immunity over time pose significant challenges to the vaccine strategy. Additionally, every medication carries potential side effects, and a "magic bullet" cure for SARS-CoV-2 currently remains elusive. Emerging evidence highlights concerning trends in the viral ability to evade and weaken the immune system. Therefore, we must broaden our approach and utilize additional, existing tools, such as quality masks, improved indoor air quality, and ventilation. The collective response to this pandemic, including public health measures and media coverage, has been uneven, with prevention efforts often falling short. This chapter aims to enlighten readers on the need for comprehensive preventive measures to protect ourselves and our communities.

Some key highlights of this chapter:

1. Understanding the life cycle of SARS-CoV-2 is crucial for developing prevention and treatment strategies. Masks can help prevent initial attachment and infection.
2. The fewer human hosts SARS-CoV-2 infects, the less likely it is to mutate and potentially outpace existing vaccines and treatments.
3. SARS-CoV-2 binds to the ACE2 receptors on the cell surface, and the ACE2 receptors are ubiquitous throughout the human body.
4. Herd immunity does not work. The endless mutation and recombination of SARS-CoV-2, and the viral persistence of SARS-CoV-2 would make it impossible for herd immunity to work.
5. A vaccine-only strategy is not enough to contain the rapidly mutating SARS-CoV-2, as vaccines effective against one strain might not work against another.
6. It's theoretically impossible that SARS-CoV-2 will mutate itself to extinction
7. SARS-CoV-2 uses ribosomes to make copies of itself, while mRNA vaccines use ribosomes to create copies of just the spike protein to train our immune system to recognize and fight the virus.
8. Paxlovid is a tool in the fight against COVID-19, but not a

magic bullet.
9. While COVID-19 rebound after Paxlovid is possible, consult your healthcare provider if concerned for personalized advice, and remember to isolate and retest if needed.
10. Paxlovid is currently unavailable for children under 12 years old or children 12 years and older who weigh less than 88 pounds. This is a serious concern, as children are at risk of developing long COVID and serious complications from COVID-19, including hospitalization and death.
11. Relying solely on vaccines, medications, and natural immunity to stop the COVID-19 pandemic is insufficient. We need to think outside the box and utilize additional existing tools, including quality masks, clean indoor air quality, and ventilation.

CHAPTER 4

Long COVID: More Than Just a Cough

~~~
*"Some wounds heal, but the scars remain." - Chinese Proverb*
~~~

COVID-19 is more than just a cough: Long COVID, also known as post-acute sequelae of COVID-19 (PASC), is a complex condition where symptoms persist or develop weeks, months, or even years after a COVID-19 infection. While a cough is a common symptom of COVID-19, many people experience far more serious effects. The virus can enter human cells via ACE-2 receptors found throughout the body, including the brain, heart, lungs, intestinal tract, pancreas, kidneys, and blood vessels.[1] Hence, the virus can affect various body organs and systems, and symptoms vary widely from person to person.

Accumulated risk of developing long COVID with each infection: Each COVID-19 infection, even mild ones, raises the risk of developing long COVID. Diseases such as hepatitis C, HIV, and Lyme disease, can initially present with "mild" symptoms similar to the flu. However, these diseases can progress to cause serious lifelong health problems, such as liver damage, AIDS, and neurological disorders. Long COVID is a debilitating illness affecting at least 10% of those infected. With over 200 symptoms ranging from fatigue to organ damage, it's a complex condition that shouldn't be treated lightly. With each reinfection, the risk of developing long COVID compounds, so prevention is crucial.[2]

Complex recovery for long COVID: There's no single cure for long COVID. Many treatment options aim to manage specific symptoms and improve quality of life. This might involve physical therapy, medication, and support groups. Remember, recovery can be slow and requires patience and understanding from both individuals and their support systems.

This chapter aims to cover some aspects of long COVID and equip you with accurate information that may not be available in mainstream media so that you can make informed decisions. Long COVID can affect anyone close to us, from family members to friends. By understanding the risks and consequences, we can encourage preventive measures. Remember, the best way to avoid long COVID is to avoid contracting COVID-19.

COVID-19's lasting shadow: The chronic reality of long COVID

The scars of the pandemic remain. COVID-19's legacy persists, impacting millions beyond the acute phase. The reality is the virus continues to claim lives and infect individuals. Even more concerning is the growing body of evidence on long COVID, a chronic condition affecting an estimated 5.3% of US adults, roughly 14 million people as of October 2023.[3] This number is likely an underestimation and is anticipated to rise further.

Long COVID can leave lasting and debilitating effects on multiple organs, potentially for years. The February 2023 Centers for Disease Control and Prevention (CDC) document "Guidance for Certifying Deaths Due to Coronavirus Disease" poignantly states: "Emerging evidence suggests that SARS-CoV-2, the virus that causes COVID-19, can have lasting effects on nearly every organ and organ system of the body weeks, months, and potentially years after infection."[4] This statement underscores that COVID-19 is both an acute and chronic disease, with acute hospitalizations and deaths alongside potential long-term health consequences like long COVID. Long COVID is not simply a prolonged illness; it's a spectrum of new or recurring symptoms impacting various body systems, ranging from fatigue and shortness of breath to brain fog and muscle aches. Its unpredictability and difficulty in diagnosis and treatment further complicate matters.

Despite this critical information, the mainstream media has largely moved on, leaving the public inadequately informed about the ongoing threat. As a result, society is operating under the misconception that COVID is a thing of the past, potentially exposing millions to unnecessary risk of developing long COVID with repeated infections.

COVID-19 and brain infection: Brain cells and skull bone marrow

While COVID-19 initially seemed to be solely a respiratory illness, research unveils that the SARS-CoV-2 virus directly infects the brain, leading to neurological complications. The key? ACE2 receptors, which are present on the surface of brain cells and act as entry points. Once inside the cells, the virus can replicate, damaging brain cells and triggering inflammation. This inflammatory response weakens the blood-brain barrier, a protective shield guarding the brain from harmful substances.[5]

The research takes the story further. The virus also targets the skull bone marrow, a site crucial for white and red blood cell production. Researchers discovered that the SARS-CoV-2 spike protein, which is part of the virus that causes COVID-19, can accumulate in the skull bone marrow, meninges, and brain tissue. The researchers studied this in mice and in tissue samples from people who had died from COVID-19. They found that the spike protein could build up in these areas and that the virus could directly kill brain cells, thereby causing brain damage and inflammation. This discovery suggests the skull bone marrow could be a "viral reservoir," potentially explaining the diverse and persistent neurological symptoms seen in some COVID-19 cases, including brain fog, headaches, fatigue, depression, and even strokes.[5]

COVID-19 and brain infection: Brain cell fusion

Researchers at Macquarie University conducted a groundbreaking study on the potential link between COVID-19 and dementia. Using innovative lab techniques, they created mini-brains from human stem cells and exposed them to the virus to investigate the effects of COVID-19 on brain function.

The study revealed a concerning finding: COVID-19 could trigger the fusion of brain cells. A possible explanation is that the virus's spike protein might act as a bridge, fusing infected cells to surrounding cells with ACE2 receptors. This "syncytial" property, where cells merge like puzzle pieces, is similar to that observed in some other viruses like the respiratory syncytial virus (RSV). This fusion, according to the research, could explain various long-term neurological symptoms including brain fog, headaches, and altered taste and smell. Additionally, the study proposes that the fused brain cells might act as a hiding place for the virus, thereby allowing the virus to evade the immune system, potentially contributing to the prolonged presence of SARS-CoV-2 in the brains of individuals with long COVID.[6]

Furthermore, the fused cells have compromised neuronal activity and die prematurely due to disrupted functionality, potentially contributing to permanent brain damage. This raises concerns about the long-term cognitive effects of COVID-19, including a potential link to dementia development.[6]

COVID-19 and the lungs: A concerning trend

The lungs, our remarkable breathtaking powerhouses, are vulnerable to COVID-19. The virus, SARS-CoV-2, gains entry into lung cells through ACE-2 receptors and can inflict significant damage. Research suggests a worrying trend: patients with COVID-19, especially those with severe infections or reinfections, face a heightened risk of developing various respiratory diseases like asthma, chronic obstructive pulmonary disease (COPD), and others. Compared to individuals with only one infection, those experiencing repeated COVID-19 infections are more susceptible to these long-term lung complications.[7]

While breathing appears effortless, it's a complex process orchestrated by our remarkable lungs. Oxygen from inhaled air seamlessly diffuses across thin alveolar walls into the bloodstream, while carbon dioxide, a waste product, travels in the opposite direction. Maintaining healthy lungs is critical for overall well-being.

Fortunately, we have measures in place to protect lung health, such as bans on indoor smoking and regulations on air pollution from factories and vehicles. However, a crucial gap exists: we lack similar legal safeguards against the acute and chronic health risks posed by airborne diseases like COVID-19, particularly in indoor spaces. This begs the question: shouldn't we consider additional measures to protect people from respiratory illnesses like COVID-19 in indoor settings?

COVID-19 and blood vessel damage: Risk of blood clots

SARS-CoV-2 binds to ACE2 receptors, which are abundant in the lining of blood vessels, heart muscle cells, and kidney cells. Imagine your body's blood vessels as a complex network of roads and highways delivering oxygen and nutrients throughout the body. Studies have shown that SARS-CoV-2 can wreak havoc on these vital pathways, increasing the risk of blood clots.[2,8] Think of the virus as causing potholes and cracks in the roads, slowing down blood flow and creating areas where clots can form like traffic jams. These clots can be very dangerous, potentially harming multiple organs.

Here are some of the potentially serious consequences of blood vessel damage caused by COVID-19:

- **Deep vein thrombosis**: Clots form deep in the legs, which can be very painful and become dangerous if they break loose and travel to the lungs or brain.
- **Pulmonary embolism**: Clots travel to the lungs, blocking blood flow and potentially causing difficulty breathing and even death.
- **Stroke**: Clots block blood flow to the brain, leading to potential brain damage, loss of function, and even death.
- **Heart failure and cardiac arrest**: Damage to blood vessels and clotting issues can put a strain on the heart, leading to heart failure or even cardiac arrest, where the heart stops functioning altogether.

The virus can also directly attack organs with many blood vessels, like the kidneys. This can damage the tiny filters within the kidneys, causing them to leak protein and blood into the urine – a sign of potential kidney problems.[8]

Researchers revealed that COVID-19 infection damages the retina, the light-sensitive tissue at the back of the eye. Damage to the tiny blood vessels in the retina may be permanent and could potentially be used as a way to assess the severity of a COVID-19 infection and predict potential long-term complications.[9]

Understanding these risks associated with COVID-19 and blood vessel damage highlights the importance of preventing infection and seeking medical attention if you experience any symptoms.

COVID-19 and the immune system: Our penetrable shield

Lymphopenia, a condition characterized by a low white blood cell count, is often associated with COVID-19. Reduced white blood cell count lowers infection-fighting capacity. The Merck Manual, a reputable medical reference, lists COVID-19 alongside HIV as one of the most common causes of acquired lymphopenia. Research shows 35% to 83% of COVID-19 patients experience lymphopenia.[10] They are more likely to require intensive care admission and have a higher risk of death due to the weakened immune system's struggle against the virus.[11] The concept of immune system weakening is relevant to both HIV and COVID-19. In both situations, the body's ability to fight off infections is significantly compromised, making individuals more susceptible to opportunistic infections and other health complications.

Additionally, research shows SARS-CoV-2 can infect and damage T cells, crucial white blood cells for fighting infections.[12] T cells help to fight off infections by recognizing and attacking foreign invaders, including viruses. Infected T cells may carry the virus throughout the body, potentially causing additional organ damage. Damaged T cells can make it more difficult for the body to fight off infections. This can lead to more severe disease and a higher risk of death. Repeated COVID-19 infections, coupled with the virus's potential to impair the immune system, raise concerns about potential long-term harm to human health.[13] Furthermore, T cells play a crucial role in the immune system's ability to identify and eliminate abnormal cells, including cancerous ones. A decrease in T cells can weaken the immune system's ability to control cancer cell growth, potentially increasing the risk of cancer development.[14]

Imagine your immune system as a shield protecting you from various illnesses. Each time you fight off an infection, like COVID-19, the shield weakens slightly. While you might still feel healthy after one or two infections, repeated encounters can significantly weaken the shield, making it harder to fight future infections. This can lead to several consequences:

- **Increased risk of severe illness**: With a weakened shield, you're more susceptible to experiencing severe complications from future COVID-19 infections.
- **Greater vulnerability to cancer and other infections**: The weakened shield might make you more susceptible to cancer and other illnesses, like bacterial, viral, or fungal infections.
- **Slower recovery times**: Fighting off infections might take longer as your immune system has less capacity.

It's important to remember that everyone's immune system is different. Older adults and those with weakened immune systems may have weaker shields from the start. Young children's immune systems are still developing, which means they may be more susceptible to infections than adults. By taking steps to prevent the spread of COVID-19, we can protect everyone, especially those most vulnerable, including young children, elderly individuals, and people with compromised immune systems.

Long COVID and postural orthostatic tachycardia syndrome (POTS):

One of the potential complications associated with long COVID is POTS.[15] POTS is a condition affecting the autonomic nervous system, which regulates involuntary functions like heart rate and blood pressure. Individuals with POTS experience an abnormal increase in heart rate (tachycardia) upon standing from a sitting or lying position, accompanied by symptoms like dizziness, lightheadedness, and fatigue.

Some possible mechanisms by which COVID-19 may cause POTS include:

- **Direct viral damage**: The virus itself could damage the autonomic nervous system, leading to POTS symptoms like irregular heart rate and blood pressure fluctuations.
- **Immune response**: The body's immune response to the virus may cause inflammation. Persistent inflammation, a common feature of long COVID, could contribute to POTS by affecting blood vessel function and nervous system communication.
- **Autoimmune reaction**: The virus may trigger an autoimmune response where the immune system attacks healthy tissues, including those involved in regulating blood pressure and heart rate.

Neither long COVID nor POTS currently has a definitive cure. However, management strategies including both pharmacological and non-pharmacological approaches can offer symptomatic relief. Diagnosing POTS in long COVID patients can be challenging due to overlapping symptoms like fatigue and dizziness. Therefore, recognizing this potential complication is crucial for accurate diagnosis and effective treatment.

Long COVID and myalgic encephalomyelitis/chronic fatigue syndrome (ME/CFS)

COVID-19 can leave lasting effects on some individuals, so it's crucial to understand the link between long COVID and ME/CFS. The term "myalgic" in ME/CFS likely stems from the Greek words "myo" meaning muscle and "algia" meaning pain, suggesting muscle pain is a potential symptom. Similarly, "encephalomyelitis" comes from "encephalo" for the brain, "myelo" for the spinal cord, and "itis" for inflammation, implying inflammation in the brain and spinal cord. ME/CFS is a long-term illness characterized by debilitating fatigue, often accompanied by muscle and joint pain, cognitive issues, and sleep problems. The cause of ME/CFS remains elusive, but genetic and environmental factors are likely contributors. Emerging evidence suggests that viral infections like COVID-19 may trigger ME/CFS symptoms in some individuals.[16]

Both long COVID and ME/CFS share a significant overlap in symptoms, making diagnosis challenging at times. This overlap includes debilitating fatigue, poor appetite, and post-exertional malaise (worsening of symptoms after exertion). Additionally, some individuals may experience a range of other symptoms, including headaches, palpitations, sleep disturbances, breathlessness, cognitive difficulties, chills, attention problems, cough, secondary depression and anxiety, reduced activity levels, muscle pain and weakness, and fluctuations in body temperature.[17]

Some possible mechanisms by which COVID-19 may trigger ME/CFS include:

- **Direct viral damage**: The virus itself could potentially damage the body's systems, leading to fatigue and other symptoms.

- **Immune response**: The body's immune response to the virus may cause inflammation, contributing to fatigue and other symptoms.
- **Autoimmune reaction**: In some cases, the virus may trigger an autoimmune response where the immune system attacks healthy cells, leading to fatigue and other symptoms.

While there is no cure for ME/CFS, there are various treatment options that can help manage symptoms:

- **Rest**: Individuals with ME/CFS often require more rest than others.
- **Pacing**: Learning to pace activities to avoid overexertion and worsening symptoms is crucial.
- **Medications**: Medications like pain relievers, antidepressants, and sleep aids can help manage specific symptoms.
- **Therapy**: Therapy can provide support in coping with the emotional and physical challenges of ME/CFS.

Millions of people around the world are now living with long COVID, which is characterized by a constellation of symptoms that can persist for months or even years after the initial COVID-19 infection. These symptoms can significantly impact a person's quality of life, making it difficult to work, attend school, or even take care of themselves. People with long COVID are often left to manage their symptoms on their own, which can be a frustrating and isolating experience.

Recognizing long COVID as a form of ME/CFS could help to improve patient care and research efforts. ME/CFS is a recognized medical condition with established diagnostic criteria and treatment protocols. By recognizing long COVID as a form of

ME/CFS, we could leverage the existing knowledge and resources to better support people with this condition.

What is the probability of getting long COVID after repeated infection?

Research suggests a significant portion of the population experiences lingering health issues following COVID-19 infection. A May 2022 CDC study reported that one in five adults (20%) aged 18 and older exhibit at least one potential long COVID symptom, rising to one in four (25%) among those 65 and older. These conditions, categorized under the term "post-acute sequelae of COVID-19" (PASC), encompass various issues like kidney complications, blood clots, respiratory and heart problems, mental health concerns, neurological issues, and musculoskeletal conditions.[18]

While the provided 20% prevalence can be used as a reference point, it's important to remember that the exact probability of getting long COVID is complex and not solely dependent on the number of infections. However, if we simplify the scenario and assume independence between infections, we can approximate the probability of developing long COVID in a healthy young adult. If we assume that there is a 20% chance of developing long COVID with each infection, then the probability of developing long COVID after repeated infection can be calculated using the following equations:

$$P\ (not\ developing\ long\ COVID) = (1 - 0.2)^x$$
$$P\ (developing\ long\ COVID) = 1 - (1 - 0.2)^x$$

where P stands for probability, x is the number of infections, and 0.2 is the 20% chance of developing long COVID. As the number of infections increases, the probability of developing long COVID increases. For example, the probability of not developing long COVID after two infections is:

$$P \text{ (not developing long COVID)} = (1 - 0.2)^2 = 0.64$$

This means that there is a 64% chance of not developing long COVID after two infections.

The probability of developing long COVID after two infections is:

$$P \text{ (developing long COVID)} = 1 - (1 - 0.2)^2 = 0.36$$

In other words, there is a 36% chance of developing long COVID after two infections.

Based on this formula, there is approximately a 59% chance of developing long COVID after four infections, and approximately an 87% chance of developing long COVID after nine infections.

It is important to note that these are just estimates, and the actual probability of developing long COVID after repeated infection varies depending on many factors including individual health, age, socioeconomic status, and variant strain. It is also important to note that long COVID is a complex condition, and the symptoms can vary from person to person. Remember, by protecting yourself from COVID-19 reinfection, you can significantly reduce your risk of developing long COVID and its associated complications.

Long COVID: A serious reality we must address

Long COVID is a real and concerning condition that can have lasting health effects for many individuals. It's not caused by psychological factors, and symptoms like fatigue, shortness of breath, and brain fog can significantly impact daily life, making it difficult to work, socialize, and participate in everyday activities.

The continued spread of COVID-19 not only strains healthcare systems and disrupts society, but also leaves many individuals with long-term health consequences. Implementing additional preventive measures like wearing quality masks, improving indoor air quality, and enhancing ventilation can significantly reduce virus transmission and its harmful effects.

Ignoring the realities of long COVID and the ongoing presence of the virus puts everyone at risk. We must raise awareness about the potential long-term consequences of COVID-19 infection and advocate for continued vigilance in infection control measures. By taking these steps, we can protect ourselves and our communities from the lasting shadow of this pandemic. Remember, prevention is key: The best way to avoid long COVID is to avoid contracting COVID-19.

Some key highlights of this chapter:

1. Long COVID is a complex condition where symptoms persist or develop weeks, months, or even years after a COVID-19 infection.
2. Long COVID can affect nearly every organ and organ system, and symptoms vary widely from person to person.
3. With each COVID-19 reinfection, the risk of developing long COVID compounds, so prevention is crucial.
4. SARS-CoV-2 can accumulate in the skull bone marrow, meninges, and brain tissue, as well as cause brain cell fusion, potentially explaining the diverse and persistent neurological symptoms of long COVID, including brain fog,

headaches, fatigue, depression, altered taste and smell, strokes, and dementia.
5. Survivors of severe COVID-19 and those facing repeat infections have increased susceptibility to developing various respiratory ailments, including asthma and COPD.
6. SARS-CoV-2 can damage blood vessels and increase the formation of blood clots. These clots can be very dangerous and travel to organs like the lungs and brain, causing serious health problems.
7. Repeated COVID-19 infections have the potential to compromise the immune system, leading to increased susceptibility to severe illness, cancer development, and other infections, as well as prolonged recovery periods.
8. Long COVID can potentially lead to POTS, a condition causing abnormal heart rate increase and dizziness upon standing.
9. Long COVID can potentially trigger symptoms resembling ME/CFS, including debilitating fatigue, muscle and joint pain, cognitive difficulties, sleep disturbances, and post-exertional malaise.
10. There's no single cure for long COVID. Many treatment options aim to manage specific symptoms and improve quality of life.
11. Prevention is key: The best way to avoid long COVID is to avoid contracting COVID-19.

PART III

PROTECTING YOURSELF, YOUR LOVED ONES, AND YOUR COMMUNITY

CHAPTER 5

Masking: Beyond Individual Choice

~~
"An ounce of prevention is worth a pound of cure."
- Benjamin Franklin
~~

The power of masks in preventing airborne transmission: The COVID-19 pandemic has shone a light on the vital role public health measures play in protecting our communities. One such measure, well-fitted, high-quality masks, has been demonstrably effective in preventing and slowing the spread of airborne viruses, including COVID-19. They are a readily available and cost-effective tool for preventing the spread of illness. However, the path to effective pandemic control has been obstructed by the spread of misinformation and politicization surrounding masks. This misinformation has had tragic consequences, costing countless lives, driving mass disablement, and leaving lasting scars on loved ones. The human cost of this misinformation cannot be ignored.

Together, we can protect ourselves and our community: Wearing a mask is a personal choice with a significant collective benefit. By making this responsible choice, we contribute to the health and well-being of our community. This connection between individual action and collective well-being is crucial in controlling the spread of airborne illnesses. Masking together strengthens our collective defense against these threats. Masks are an effective tool when used correctly, and they complement other preventive measures like hand hygiene and social distancing to create a multi-layered approach to protecting ourselves and others.

The spread of misinformation can be harmful and create a false sense of security. To empower informed action, we will address some common misinformation about masking:

- Misinformation: Masks don't work against COVID-19.
- Misinformation: Cloth masks are sufficient protection against COVID-19.
- Misinformation: Viruses are too small for masks to block.
- Misinformation: Masks are unnecessary outdoors.
- Misinformation: Masks cause low oxygen levels.
- Misinformation: Other measures like hand hygiene, distancing, and sanitizing are enough.

Additionally, we will explore other aspects of masking, including cultural contexts and practices of masking in different countries, as well as the ethical implications. By understanding how masks work, addressing misinformation, and embracing our shared responsibility, we can collectively build a stronger defense against airborne transmission and protect the health of our community.

Misinformation: Masks don't work against COVID-19.

Masks are a crucial tool in our arsenal against airborne viruses like COVID-19. Studies found that wearing face masks in public spaces reduces the spread of COVID-19. Counties with a mask mandate had a decrease in COVID-19 cases, while counties without a mask mandate continued to see an increase. These findings highlight the potential of mask mandates in mitigating the spread of the virus and protecting public health.[1,2] It is important that everyone wears masks in public, not just healthcare workers.

This is because masks can help prevent people who are sick from spreading the virus to others. Thus, masks help to control hospital and community transmissions.[3]

There are two main ways that masks prevent the spread of COVID-19:

1. **Filtration**: Masks can filter out respiratory droplets and aerosols that are produced when one coughs, sneezes, or talks. This filtration is most effective with masks made of multiple layers of fabric and a special material designed to block particles as small as 0.3 micrometers in size. Masks rated as P100, N100, N95, KN95, or KF94 indicate the filtration efficiency, with P100 and N100 offering the highest protection (at 99.97%), followed by N95 and KN95 (95%), and KF94 (94%).
2. **Physical barrier**: Masks can also act as a physical barrier that prevents respiratory droplets from reaching others. This is especially effective with masks that fit snugly over your nose and mouth.

The effectiveness of well-fitted, high-quality masks in preventing airborne transmission of viruses, including COVID-19, is indisputable.

Misinformation: Cloth masks are sufficient protection against COVID-19.

The effectiveness of masks at blocking respiratory droplets and aerosols depends on the type of mask, the fit of the mask, and the size of the airborne particles.

- P100 or N100 respirators are the most effective at blocking respiratory droplets and aerosols. They can filter out 99.97% of airborne particles.
- N95 and KN95 respirators are effective as well, and they can filter out 95% of airborne particles, including aerosols.
- Surgical masks are less effective than N95 respirators at filtering out aerosols.
- Cloth masks are the least effective at filtering out aerosols.

N95 and KN95 masks, as well as other high-quality masks, are highly effective in blocking airborne particles from reaching your airways. Surgical and cloth masks offer less protection, and their effectiveness depends on the number of layers, the materials used, and how well they fit.[4] It is important to note that the effectiveness of masks in reducing the risk of infection depends on numerous factors, including the type of mask, the fit of the mask, and the wearer's behavior.

Additionally, here are some other things to keep in mind when wearing a mask:

- Wash your hands before and after putting on and taking off your mask.
- Make sure the mask fits snugly over your nose and mouth.
- Avoid touching your face while you are wearing the mask.
- Replace your mask if it becomes wet or soiled.

By following these simple tips, you can help protect yourself and others from the spread of COVID-19.

Misinformation: Viruses are too small for masks to block.

While SARS-CoV-2 measures around 0.1 micrometers, it doesn't travel alone. It hitches a ride on respiratory droplets and aerosols, which are much larger and easily blocked by high-quality masks.[5] Here is a quick summary of the types of respiratory particles:

- **Droplets**: Droplets are produced when a person breathes, coughs, sneezes, speaks, sings, or exercises. These droplets have a diameter of 5 micrometers or greater and can contain viruses that cause infection. Larger droplets can fall to the ground within seconds, while smaller droplets can stay suspended in the air for longer periods.
- **Aerosols**: Aerosols are created when respiratory droplets evaporate. These aerosols have a diameter of less than 5 micrometers and can also contain viruses that cause infection. They can remain suspended in the air for much longer and travel long distances, increasing the risk of inhalation.

Masks wearing helps to reduce the risk of infection in two ways:

- **Block droplets and aerosols**: Well-fitting, high-quality masks like N95 and KN95 utilize a series of electrostatic and mechanical filtration mechanisms. These filters are composed of materials with intricate structures designed to block airborne particles, including respiratory droplets and aerosols.
- **Reduce emission**: Masks also reduce the overall amount of droplets and aerosols expelled, further minimizing the risk of transmission.

Infection is not a one-dimensional equation. It is a complex interplay between various factors:

- **Infectivity of the individual**: This includes the amount of virus they shed through coughing, sneezing, or exhaling.
- **Viral load in the environment**: This depends on the number of infected individuals present and the

concentration of airborne droplets and aerosols containing the virus.
- **Environmental factors**: These include wind speed, wind direction, humidity, ventilation, and crowd density, all impacting viral spread.
- **Exposure duration and intensity**: Longer exposure to higher concentrations of the virus increases the risk of infection.

Understanding these factors empowers us to make informed choices to protect ourselves and others, like wearing masks which can significantly reduce exposure to airborne viruses and minimize the risk of infection.

Misinformation: Masks are unnecessary outdoors.

Outdoor spaces offer a lower risk of COVID-19 transmission compared to indoors. However, complete safety isn't guaranteed and infection remains possible due to the airborne nature of the virus. Respiratory droplets and aerosols containing the virus are expelled when an infected person coughs, sneezes, talks, or exhales. While droplets settle quickly, aerosols can linger in the air for longer durations, potentially traveling further distances. The risk of infection increases in crowded outdoor settings or when individuals are in close proximity.

A study in China investigated a super-spreading event of the SARS-CoV-2 virus at an outdoor night market. The researchers discovered that aerosols containing the virus can remain infectious for up to 1 hour and 39 minutes within the open-air environment. This finding suggests that aerosols can potentially transmit the virus over longer distances, even outdoors.[6]

Similar to how cigarette smoke can linger in the air, COVID-19, like many respiratory illnesses, can linger in the air through tiny airborne particles called aerosols. These microscopic particles are invisible to the naked eye and can carry the virus, lingering in the air for extended periods and potentially being inhaled by others. Additionally, when wind speed is low, virus particles may linger in the air for longer, increasing the risk of infection during unmasked social gatherings outdoors. While the risk of infection is generally lower outdoors compared to indoors, it can still occur, especially in crowded settings or close contact situations. Wearing a well-fitting, high-quality mask in these situations can offer additional protection.

Misinformation: Masks cause low oxygen levels.

In the ongoing fight against misinformation surrounding COVID-19, one persistent claim asserts that wearing masks leads to dangerously low oxygen levels. This claim, however, is entirely false and misleading. Masks are designed from breathable fabrics that allow for sufficient air exchange. Studies have demonstrated that wearing surgical or N95 masks does not cause a decrease in blood oxygen saturation, supporting their safety and effectiveness in preventing the spread of COVID-19.[7,8]

While masks are safe and effective in preventing the spread of COVID-19, they might feel slightly uncomfortable for some people, especially during physical exertion. This discomfort can stem from:

- Increased humidity and warmth are trapped within the mask, leading to a feeling of breathlessness.
- Psychological factors including anxiety or claustrophobia can be exacerbated by the sensation of wearing a mask.

Here are some tips for making mask wearing more comfortable:

- **Mask fit**: A poorly fitted mask can cause discomfort by rubbing against the face or leaking air around the edges. Choosing the right size and fit can significantly improve comfort.
- **Oral hygiene**: Maintaining good oral hygiene, including brushing at least twice daily, flossing and tongue scraping regularly, and addressing underlying dental issues, is crucial for fresh breath and overall health, making mask wearing more comfortable.

Wearing masks is a safe and effective way to prevent the spread of COVID-19. They do not cause low oxygen levels in healthy individuals and are crucial in protecting both yourself and others from the virus.

Misinformation: Other measures like hand hygiene, distancing, and sanitizing are enough.

While hand hygiene, distancing, and sanitizing are crucial strategies in combating COVID-19, they are not enough on their own when the virus is airborne.

Public health measures, like washing hands, maintaining physical distance, and disinfecting surfaces, are essential practices. However, these are most effective when combined with mask-wearing to address the leading mode of transmission: airborne respiratory droplets and aerosols.

Wearing a well-fitting, high-quality mask, like an N95 or KN95 respirator, significantly reduces your risk of inhaling these virus-laden particles. This additional layer of protection helps to safeguard both yourself and others from COVID-19 infection.

Masking practices around the world: Individual choice vs. collective responsibility

Mask wearing has become ingrained in certain cultures around the globe. The benefits of masking extend beyond just preventing the spread of illness. Masks can act as filters, reducing exposure to dust, pollen, and other airborne irritants, thereby improving breathing comfort, particularly for those with allergies or sensitivities.

In places including Taiwan and Japan, wearing a mask is seen as a demonstration of consideration, respect for others, and social responsibility. It signifies awareness of the potential to spread illness, a commitment to self-care, and a desire to protect the community.

However, it's important to understand that the perception of masking varies significantly across cultures. In some countries, mask wearing might be viewed primarily as a personal health choice. While respecting individual preferences is crucial, it's equally important to encourage collective responsibility in mitigating the spread of airborne diseases.

It's important to remember that true freedom thrives in a society where individual liberties are balanced with consideration for others. While individual choice is a cornerstone of a healthy society, it doesn't give us the right to disregard the potential consequences of our actions on the health and well-being of those around us. This approach to masking goes beyond obligation. It represents an understanding of shared responsibility and a willingness to take proactive steps for collective well-being.

Therefore, fostering a culture of mutual respect and collective responsibility is crucial. By promoting evidence-based information and encouraging compassionate communication, we can create a society where individuals understand the impact of their choices and are empowered to protect both themselves and their communities.

Why masks make sense in the fight against COVID-19

Wearing a mask is a simple yet highly effective way to protect yourself and others from COVID-19.

Why should you wear a mask?

- **Reduced transmission**: Masks create a physical barrier that blocks respiratory droplets and aerosols containing the virus from being expelled when you cough, sneeze, or even talk. This significantly reduces the risk of you spreading the virus to others, even if you are asymptomatic.
- **Protection for yourself**: While not 100% foolproof, masks can also offer some level of protection against inhaling infected respiratory droplets and aerosols expelled by others.
- **Complements other measures**: Masking works best alongside other preventive measures including ventilation, social distancing, and hand hygiene. It forms a crucial layer of defense in mitigating the spread of the virus.

The opportunity cost of masking:

- **Minor discomfort**: Wearing a mask can cause some discomfort, especially during hot weather or physical exertion. However, using well-fitting, breathable masks can significantly mitigate this.
- **Social interaction**: Masks can slightly impede communication, particularly facial expressions. However,

with practice, most people adapt effectively, and the benefits far outweigh this minor inconvenience.

The opportunity cost of NOT masking:

- **Increased risk of infection**: Not masking significantly increases your risk of contracting and spreading COVID-19, especially in crowded settings or when interacting with individuals of unknown COVID-19 status.
- **Potential for severe illness and long-term complications**: COVID-19 can lead to severe illness, hospitalization, and even death, even in young, healthy individuals. It can also cause long COVID affecting various organs and systems.
- **Strain on healthcare systems**: A surge in infections due to not masking can put immense strain on healthcare resources, limiting access to critical care for other needs.

Additionally, wearing a mask is an action grounded in strong ethical values, and it is the right thing to do. Here are some key principles at play:

- **Empathy and compassion**: Choosing to wear a mask demonstrates our empathy and compassion. It safeguards the vulnerable from potential illness, embodying the Golden Rule's message of treating others as we wish to be treated.
- **Collective responsibility**: Public health thrives on collective action. By wearing a mask, we acknowledge that individual choices can significantly impact the health and safety of our entire community. This simple act of shared responsibility empowers us to become stewards of public well-being.
- **Protecting the vulnerable**: Individuals with compromised immune systems, the elderly, or those with underlying

health conditions often face heightened risks from infectious diseases. Wearing a mask minimizes the possibility of unknowingly transmitting illness and demonstrates respect for their vulnerabilities.
- **Respect for healthcare workers**: By reducing the spread of infection, masking alleviates the burden on healthcare professionals already stretched thin. It shows respect for their efforts and helps preserve their health and capacity to care for others.

While wearing a mask may involve some minor inconveniences, the benefits far outweigh them. This simple act protects both yourself and others, preventing serious illness and contributing to managing the pandemic. Remember, masking isn't just about individual protection; it's a collective act of responsibility for our communities and healthcare systems.

Overcoming the fear of judgment when masking

While concerns about judgment are understandable, remember that protecting your health and the health of others far outweighs any potential negativity. Wearing a mask is a responsible and selfless act, demonstrating your commitment to the well-being of everyone around you, including those who may be more vulnerable to illness.

Here are some additional points to consider:

- **Challenge negative thoughts:** When faced with self-doubt, challenge it with logic. Are the opinions of misinformed individuals about your mask worth risking the health of your family and others?

- **Focus on the positive impact:** Wearing a mask demonstrates your care and respect for yourself and others. You are prioritizing health and safety.
- **Practice self-compassion:** Acknowledge your fear of judgment, but don't let it control your actions. Remind yourself that your decision to wear a mask is based on evidence and care, not fear of others' opinions.
- **Many people support masking:** You are not alone in choosing to protect yourself and others. A significant portion of the population encourages responsible behavior like mask wearing.
- **Misinformed opinions don't define you or your values:** Focus on what truly matters – your health, the health of your loved ones, and contributing to a safer community.

By focusing on the bigger picture, the positive impact you make, and prioritizing your well-being, you can overcome the fear of judgment and remain confident in your decision to wear a mask. Remember, your health and the health of others matter most.

Some key highlights of this chapter:

1. By wearing masks in public spaces, we significantly reduce the spread of COVID-19 through airborne transmission. This vital step helps control the spread in hospitals and communities, ultimately protecting everyone.
2. N95 and KN95 respirators, as well as other high-quality respirators, provide enhanced protection against airborne particles compared to surgical and cloth masks.
3. SARS-CoV-2 primarily spreads through respiratory droplets and aerosols. These particles can be effectively blocked by well-fitting, high-quality masks.
4. While outdoor transmission of COVID-19 is generally considered lower than indoors, it can still occur, especially

in crowded settings or close contact situations. Wearing a well-fitting, high-quality mask in these situations can offer additional protection.
5. Made from breathable materials, masks allow for adequate air exchange, ensuring comfort and safety. Studies confirm that wearing surgical and N95 masks doesn't significantly decrease blood oxygen levels, further supporting their effectiveness in preventing COVID-19 spread.
6. Masks are an essential layer of protection, alongside other preventive measures.
7. Wearing a mask transcends personal choice, becoming an act of responsibility, kindness, and collective action towards protecting the well-being of ourselves and the most vulnerable in our communities.

CHAPTER 6

Clean Air

~~~
*"The very first canon of nursing...: keep the air he breathes as pure as the external air, without chilling him."*
*- Florence Nightingale*
~~~

The overlooked necessity of clean air: Clean air is a fundamental human right essential for a healthy life. Yet, it remains underappreciated and underinvested in communities. While we readily acknowledge the importance of clean water and earthquake-resistant buildings, ensuring access to clean indoor air often falls short. This negligence has significant consequences for public health, contributing to the spread of airborne diseases and negatively impacting overall well-being. Just like Florence Nightingale, the pioneer of modern nursing, championed the importance of ventilation for patient recovery over 150 years ago, we must recognize the vital role it plays in our fight against airborne illnesses.

Ensuring healthier communities through investment in clean air: Current building codes, unfortunately, often fall short in guaranteeing adequate air quality and preventing the transmission of these diseases. To safeguard the health of our communities, we urgently need to update building codes. These updated codes should mandate enhanced filtration systems, clean air delivery mechanisms, and improved ventilation infrastructure. This proactive approach will ensure that buildings not only provide physical shelter but also actively contribute to the health and well-being of their occupants. By prioritizing clean air, we can create safer, healthier environments for everyone. This investment in our communities will have a lasting impact on public health, reducing the spread of airborne illnesses and fostering a healthier future for all.

This chapter unveils the silent threat of airborne diseases and the tools to combat them. We'll explore the importance of ventilation and filtration, the role of CO_2 monitors in maintaining healthy air quality, and the critical need for clean air in schools and all indoor spaces. Clean air is not a privilege, it's a fundamental right. By equipping ourselves with this knowledge, we can harness the power of improved ventilation and filtration systems to create healthier environments and significantly reduce the spread of airborne illnesses across the board.

The invisible threat of airborne transmission of disease

For millennia, the silent threat of airborne diseases has lurked among us. When people gather in poorly ventilated spaces with limited filtration, the air itself can become a carrier of microscopic hitchhikers – bacteria, viruses, and fungi. These invisible passengers can travel through the air when an infected person coughs, sneezes or even breathes, silently spreading various illnesses. Here are some common airborne diseases:

- **Viral**: The common cold, chickenpox, influenza, measles, mumps, COVID-19, and respiratory syncytial virus (RSV) are just some of the many viruses that can be transmitted through the air.

- **Bacterial**: Diseases like tuberculosis, whooping cough, and Legionnaires' disease are spread through airborne bacteria.
- **Fungal**: Fungal spores, like those from Aspergillus, can also travel through the air and cause illness.

While airborne illnesses are a significant concern, maintaining good air quality is essential for overall health. Air pollution, containing a variety of particles, can contribute to respiratory problems, heart disease, and even cancer. We can take steps to mitigate these threats and create a healthier environment. Improved ventilation in buildings allows for better air circulation, reducing the concentration of airborne particles. Filtration systems capture and remove these contaminants, further safeguarding our health. By understanding the silent threat of airborne disease and prioritizing clean air, we can create healthier spaces for ourselves and future generations.

Breathe clean air: the power of ventilation and filtration

We spend a significant amount of time indoors, whether it's at home, work, school, or public spaces. While we may not always think about it, the quality of the air we breathe indoors has a major impact on our health, comfort, and productivity. Indoor air pollution can include microscopic organisms and other harmful pollutants, posing a significant threat. However, there are two key defenses you can utilize to create a healthy indoor environment: ventilation and filtration.

Ventilation is the process of bringing in fresh outdoor air and removing stale indoor air. There are two main types:

- **Natural ventilation**: Opening windows and doors allows for natural airflow. This is a simple and cost-effective

solution, but it's weather-dependent and may not be sufficient in all climates.
- **Mechanical ventilation**: Systems like fans and air exchangers use ducts and vents to bring in fresh air and exhaust stale air continuously. This offers greater control over ventilation rates and can be integrated with heating and cooling systems for better efficiency.

Proper ventilation helps dilute and remove these pollutants by bringing in fresh outdoor air and exhausting stale indoor air. This creates a healthier and more comfortable environment for everyone inside.

Filtration works by trapping airborne pollutants using filters. Different filters target different particle sizes:

- **Minimum Efficiency Reporting Value (MERV) filters**: Common in HVAC systems, these filters have a rating that indicates how well they capture airborne particles. Higher MERV ratings trap smaller particles. However, denser filters can restrict airflow, potentially straining your HVAC system. For compatibility advice, consult your system's manual or a qualified technician.
- **High Efficiency Particulate Air (HEPA) filters**: HEPA filters can theoretically remove at least 99.97% of dust, pollen, mold, bacteria, viruses, and any airborne particles with a size of 0.3 microns.

If you're looking for a cost-effective alternative to purchasing a traditional air purifier, consider building a Corsi-Rosenthal Box. This simple yet effective design utilizes readily available materials for impressive air filtration. A box fan forms one side of the box, while the other sides are constructed using high-grade air filters, typically MERV-13 or higher. The box fan pulls air through the filters, trapping dust, allergens, and even viruses. Clean air is then expelled back into the room. Instructions and detailed plans for building your Corsi-Rosenthal Box can be easily found online.

By prioritizing ventilation and filtration, you can create a haven of clean, healthy air within your home, office, or school. Here are some steps you can take to improve your indoor air quality:

- **Increase ventilation**: Open windows regularly, especially during pleasant weather.
- **Run exhaust fans**: Use them in kitchens and bathrooms during and after use.
- **Invest in air filtration**: Consider upgrading your HVAC filters, adding portable HEPA air purifiers, or building your own Corsi-Rosenthal Box.
- **Schedule maintenance**: Ensure ventilation systems are functioning properly by having them serviced regularly and filters are replaced regularly.

Remember, a breath of fresh air is just as important indoors as it is outdoors. Take action today to create a cleaner, healthier indoor environment for yourself and those around you.

Fresh air, fewer airborne diseases: The impact of air change rate in indoor spaces

The air change rate (ACH) is a direct measure of a space's ventilation efficiency. ACH refers to the number of times the entire volume of air in a space is completely replaced with fresh outdoor air per hour. Higher ACH can significantly reduce the risk of airborne disease transmission indoors. Here's how:

- **Dilution**: Increased ACH brings in more fresh outdoor air, diluting the concentration of airborne contaminants, including viruses and bacteria. Imagine a crowded room

with little ventilation compared to a room with high ACH – it's like opening multiple windows in the high ACH room, dispersing the contaminants and reducing the risk of airborne transmission.
- **Removal**: Fresh air replaces stale air that may contain infectious particles. This helps remove these particles from the breathing zone and reduce the overall amount of airborne pathogens within the space.
- **Reduced Exposure Time**: A higher ACH shortens the time an infectious particle remains airborne. This reduces the chance of someone inhaling the particle and potentially becoming infected.

A study examining the impact of ventilation rates on airborne transmission highlights that various guidelines recommend a minimum of 12 air changes per hour (ACH) for airborne infection isolation rooms.[1] This high ACH translates to completely replacing the air in the space with fresh outdoor air approximately every five minutes. This frequent air exchange plays a crucial role in mitigating the spread of airborne diseases by diluting, removing, and reducing exposure time to airborne contaminants, making it particularly effective in high-risk settings including healthcare isolation rooms. Given the positive impact of high ACH on reducing airborne disease transmission, it's worth considering its application in high-occupancy spaces including schools, workplaces, and nursing homes.

ACH works in concert with other preventive measures like well-fitted, high-quality masks and filtration to create a layered defense against airborne contaminants, especially in crowded spaces or high-risk situations. The combined effect of these measures significantly reduces the risk of airborne disease transmission. It's like having multiple lines of defense working together to create a safer and healthier indoor environment.

Measuring air quality: The role of CO2 monitors

Humans breathe in oxygen and exhale carbon dioxide (CO2) as a waste product. Luckily, unlike Florence Nightingale's era, technology has provided us with a valuable tool to measure the amount of CO2 in the air: the CO2 monitor. The global average atmospheric CO2 concentration in 2022 was 417.06 parts per million (ppm), meaning roughly 0.04% of our air is CO2.[2]

Here's a breakdown of the gases in the air:

- Nitrogen (around 78%)
- Oxygen (around 21%)
- CO2 (around 0.04%)
- Other gases (around 1%)

While carbon dioxide only makes up about 0.04% of the air we breathe, the human body is surprisingly sensitive to even minor fluctuations in its levels. Here's why:

Hemoglobin, the iron-rich protein found in red blood cells, acts as a critical transport system within our bodies. It efficiently transports oxygen from the lungs to tissues, picking up CO2 waste products along the way and returning them to the lungs for exhalation. Hemoglobin has a decreased affinity to oxygen as CO2 levels increase, and CO2 does this in two ways:

- **The Bohr Effect**: When CO2 levels rise, it creates a more acidic environment in the blood (lower pH). This acidity triggers a change in hemoglobin, making it less willing to hold onto oxygen molecules.
- **Direct Competition**: CO2 can directly bind to a specific site on hemoglobin that's also meant for oxygen. This further reduces the available space for oxygen to bind.

The problem arises when CO2 levels in the surrounding air increase, like in a crowded, poorly ventilated room. These higher levels make hemoglobins less efficient at delivering oxygen to tissues. This can lead to a range of negative effects, including decreased cognitive function, fatigue, and headaches.

A study examined the impact of CO2 on cognitive function in simulated office environments. The findings suggest that high CO2 levels, independent of other factors, can significantly decrease cognitive abilities, potentially leading to reduced productivity and overall well-being. For instance, the study revealed that CO2 concentrations around 1000 ppm may decrease cognitive function by 15%, and CO2 concentrations around 1400 ppm may decrease cognitive function by as much as 50%.[3]

Here is a summary of CO2 levels and indoor air quality:

- Around 420 ppm: Similar to fresh outdoor air, suggesting good ventilation and sufficient oxygen.
- 500 ppm to 1000 ppm: Increasing CO2 levels, possibly due to moderate crowding or limited ventilation.
- Above 1000 ppm: Indicates poor air quality, potentially caused by inadequate ventilation or overcrowding. This may lead to drowsiness and reduced cognitive function.

Note: While CO2 levels are a useful indicator, other factors can affect air quality.

Maintaining low indoor CO2 levels is crucial for a healthy environment. Ideally, CO2 concentrations should stay below 1000 ppm, and even closer to 420 ppm, which reflects fresh outdoor air. CO2 monitors offer a valuable tool for managing indoor air quality by providing real-time feedback on ventilation. Since CO2 levels tend to rise with occupancy and limited ventilation, monitoring CO2 can help ensure sufficient fresh air is introduced to maintain a healthy and productive environment. Monitoring CO2 levels can also signal the need for increased ventilation to prevent the spread of airborne illnesses, especially in crowded areas. Using CO2 monitors would be beneficial in indoor settings, including homes, offices, schools, and healthcare facilities.

Clean air for children

Imagine this: You've poured your heart and soul into raising a healthy child. Sacrifices made, sleepless nights endured, and now they're off to school, brimming with excitement. But instead of learning and thriving, they come home sick often. Contaminated air at school is the culprit, potentially spreading illness throughout the family. This isn't just inconvenient, it's heartbreaking. Schools including daycare centers should be safe havens, and clean air is a fundamental part of that equation.

Schools play a vital role in our communities, but they can also be hubs for airborne disease transmission. With nearly half the population interacting with schools directly or indirectly, outbreaks there can quickly spread throughout the community.[4] Finding a balance between adaptation and mitigation is key. By implementing effective strategies like improved ventilation and filtration, alongside responsible mask use, we can keep schools safe havens for learning while minimizing the risk of community spread.

Protecting children from preventable illnesses remains a core responsibility. Normalizing sickness in children is not only unfair but also irresponsible, potentially leading to long-term health complications. Framing the issue as a choice between mitigation measures and children's well-being creates a false dichotomy. Children are integral parts of our communities, and their health impacts the broader population. Prioritizing clean air strategies like ventilation, filtration, and CO2 monitoring can significantly curb in-school transmission, protecting both children and the community as a whole.

The potential for long-term health effects and repeated COVID-19 infections in children is an ongoing concern.[5] Schools can prioritize student well-being by implementing strategies to minimize the spread of the virus. The success story of a Brisbane school in Queensland, Australia, in 2022 offers valuable insights. Dads at the school used science and engineering principles to improve classroom ventilation. By combining air circulation techniques, HEPA filters, and CO2 monitoring, they effectively prevented outbreaks during the Omicron wave. This example demonstrates that a multi-layered approach can significantly decrease the risk of COVID-19 transmission in schools.[6]

Maintaining clean air in schools through a combination of ventilation, filtration, and CO2 monitoring offers many benefits for students, staff, and teachers.

- **Reduced risk of illness**: Clean air significantly reduces the spread of airborne respiratory illnesses, including COVID-19, influenza, RSV, and the common cold. This translates to a healthier learning environment with fewer student, teacher, and staff absences due to illness.
- **Enhanced learning and performance**: Improved air quality and ventilation have been linked to increased cognitive function, focus, and concentration in students. This can lead to better academic performance, a more productive learning environment, and a more positive overall school experience.
- **Improved comfort and well-being**: Clean air creates a more comfortable learning environment, reducing drowsiness, headaches, and respiratory irritation. This can

lead to increased student and staff well-being, fostering a more positive and productive atmosphere.

By prioritizing clean air strategies, schools can create a healthier and more conducive learning environment for everyone. In addition to clean air strategies, encouraging well-fitting, high-quality masks and adhering to evidence-based and sensible health and safety protocols can provide further layers of defense against the spread of diseases in schools.

Clean air is a fundamental human right

Clean air is essential for a healthy life, just like clean water. Just like we wouldn't drink contaminated water from the faucets, we shouldn't be forced to breathe in contaminated air, especially indoors. Access to clean water is a fundamental human right and a public health imperative because it stops the spread of disease. Shouldn't the same principle apply to the air we breathe indoors? Absolutely. The need for collective action for clean air in indoor spaces is urgent.

Like the fight against secondhand smoke, we now face a critical decision regarding COVID-19. Just as we wouldn't tolerate secondhand smoke in public spaces anymore, we shouldn't accept compromised air quality indoors. For decades, smoking was commonplace indoors, including in doctors' offices and workplaces. However, public advocacy and decisions grounded on science eventually led to the ban on smoking indoors. Today, protecting everyone from repeated COVID-19 infections demands a similar approach.

Here's why clean air and preventative measures matter:

- **Long-term health complications**: Repeated COVID-19 infections increase the risks of developing long-term health complications.
- **Vulnerable populations**: Children, elderly, pregnant women, and those with compromised immune systems are at greater risk from COVID-19 and secondary infections.

Prioritizing clean air isn't just about protecting ourselves from COVID-19. It's an investment in our collective health, our economy, and our future. Here's why:

- **Reduced Transmission**: Proper ventilation and filtration systems in schools and public spaces can significantly reduce the spread of COVID-19 and other airborne illnesses.
- **Long-Term Health Benefits**: Clean air protects vulnerable populations and reduces the risk of long-term health complications.
- **Economic Advantages**: A healthier population means fewer sick days and increased productivity.

Investing in clean air solutions like ventilation and filtration systems, alongside appropriate mask use, can unlock a future filled with healthier lives, stronger communities, and a more sustainable world. Amazon's high-tech headquarters in Virginia serves as a compelling example. Their advanced filtration and ventilation systems constantly monitor CO_2 levels and remove harmful contaminants.[7] Imagine this technology becoming commonplace – transforming the air quality in schools, workplaces, restaurants, nursing homes, and beyond. By prioritizing clean air, we're not just safeguarding health – we're building a more resilient future for generations to come. Clean air shouldn't be a privilege; it's a fundamental right.

Some key highlights of this chapter:

1. Microscopic organisms - bacteria, viruses, and fungi - can infect a person through airborne transmission.
2. Ventilation helps dilute and remove airborne particles by bringing in fresh outdoor air and exhausting stale indoor air.
3. Filtration uses filters to trap airborne particles. Higher-rated MERV filters and HEPA filters are particularly effective at capturing these particles, including microscopic organisms.
4. High-occupancy spaces including schools, workplaces, and nursing homes should have a minimum of 12 air changes per hour.
5. Despite making up only 0.04% of inhaled air, the human body is remarkably sensitive to fluctuations in carbon dioxide levels.
6. CO_2 concentrations around 1000 ppm may decrease cognitive function by 15%, and CO_2 concentrations around 1400 ppm may decrease cognitive function by as much as 50%.
7. CO_2 monitors complement ventilation and filtration by ensuring fresh air for a healthy and productive environment.
8. Prioritizing clean air strategies like ventilation, filtration, and CO_2 monitoring can significantly curb in-school transmission, protecting both children and the community as a whole.
9. Clean air is not a privilege, it's a fundamental right. We must invest in clean air for the sake of our collective health, economy, and future.

Epilogue

A Ripple of Hope

~~~
*"I alone cannot change the world, but I can cast a stone across the waters to create many ripples."* - Mother Teresa
~~~

This journey through the book is complete, and I thank you for joining me with an open mind for positive change. Let's face it, dismantling years of misinformation takes time. Convincing someone in a few hours to question deeply held beliefs can be a tall order. That's why I wrote this book - to create a lasting resource for anyone seeking truth about airborne illnesses.

Even a single pebble tossed in a pond can cause ripples that spread outward. I believe my actions, through this book, can inspire others to create their own ripples of positive change. Remember, significant progress often begins with small steps.

Empowered to protect

By now, you're equipped to protect yourself, loved ones, and your community from COVID-19 and similar threats.

- Chapter 1 exposed the ongoing challenge of misinformation surrounding the pandemic. You've learned to distinguish factual information from media opinions.

- Chapter 2 delved into the media's role in shaping perception. This understanding empowers you to critically assess any information you encounter.

- Chapter 3 unveiled the science behind SARS-CoV-2, our common enemy. Knowing this enemy lets you see the bigger picture and leverage effective tools to fight it.

- Chapter 4 highlighted the risks of long COVID and the importance of prevention. After all, the best defense against long COVID is to avoid contracting the virus itself.

- Chapter 5 addressed common myths about masking and emphasized its effectiveness in preventing airborne transmission. You're now confident in masking because it's the right thing to do, regardless of perception.

- Chapter 6 provided practical tips on maintaining clean air indoors, empowering you to advocate for safe environments and minimize airborne transmission risks.

Together we rise

You're now equipped to make informed decisions for your well-being and advocate for positive change. Our collective well-being depends on cooperation and understanding. With this knowledge, I believe humanity can overcome the threat of airborne diseases in the years to come.

If this book resonated with you, please consider leaving a review on Amazon and recommending it to others.

Best wishes for continued health and safety.

Anton Wang

NOTES

Introduction

1. CHAN-YEUNG M, XU R. SARS: epidemiology. Respirol Carlton Vic. 2003;8(Suppl 1):S9-S14. doi:10.1046/j.1440-1843.2003.00518.x
2. Lee N, Hui D, Wu A, et al. A major outbreak of severe acute respiratory syndrome in Hong Kong. N Engl J Med. 2003;348(20):1986-1994. doi:10.1056/NEJMoa030685
3. Ge XY, Hu B, Shi ZL. Bat Coronaviruses. In: Bats and Viruses. John Wiley & Sons, Ltd; 2015:127-155. doi:10.1002/9781118818824.ch5
4. Lu R, Zhao X, Li J, et al. Genomic characterisation and epidemiology of 2019 novel coronavirus: implications for virus origins and receptor binding. The Lancet. 2020;395(10224):565-574. doi:10.1016/S0140-6736(20)30251-8
5. Kirtipal N, Bharadwaj S, Kang SG. From SARS to SARS-CoV-2, insights on structure, pathogenicity and immunity aspects of pandemic human coronaviruses. Infect Genet Evol J Mol Epidemiol Evol Genet Infect Dis. 2020;85:104502. doi:10.1016/j.meegid.2020.104502
6. Zhang XY, Huang HJ, Zhuang DL, et al. Biological, clinical and epidemiological features of COVID-19, SARS and MERS and AutoDock simulation of ACE2. Infect Dis Poverty. 2020;9(1):99. doi:10.1186/s40249-020-00691-6
7. Proal AD, VanElzakker MB. Long COVID or Post-acute Sequelae of COVID-19 (PASC): An Overview of Biological Factors That May Contribute to Persistent Symptoms. Front Microbiol. 2021;12. Accessed January 4, 2024. https://www.frontiersin.org/articles/10.3389/fmicb.2021.698169
8. Morens DM, Folkers GK, Fauci AS. The Concept of Classical Herd Immunity May Not Apply to COVID-19. J Infect Dis. 2022;226(2):195-198. doi:10.1093/infdis/jiac109

Chapter 1: Misinformation on the Characteristics of COVID-19

1. COVID-19 deaths | WHO COVID-19 dashboard. datadot. Accessed January 14, 2024. https://data.who.int/dashboards/covid19/cases
2. How many people in the US have long COVID? USAFacts.

Accessed January 14, 2024. https://usafacts.org/articles/how-many-people-have-long-covid/
3. Guidance for Certifying Deaths Due to Coronavirus Disease 2019 (COVID–19): Expanded in February 2023 to Include Guidance for Certifying Deaths Due to Post-Acute Sequelae of COVID-19. National Center for Health Statistics (U.S.); 2023. doi:10.15620/cdc:124588
4. Fears AC, Klimstra WB, Duprex P, et al. Persistence of Severe Acute Respiratory Syndrome Coronavirus 2 in Aerosol Suspensions - Volume 26, Number 9—September 2020 - Emerging Infectious Diseases journal - CDC. doi:10.3201/eid2609.201806
5. Kohanski MA, Lo LJ, Waring MS. Review of indoor aerosol generation, transport, and control in the context of COVID-19. Int Forum Allergy Rhinol. 2020;10(10):1173-1179. doi:10.1002/alr.22661
6. Miller SL, Nazaroff WW, Jimenez JL, et al. Transmission of SARS-CoV-2 by inhalation of respiratory aerosol in the Skagit Valley Chorale superspreading event. Indoor Air. 2021;31(2):314-323. doi:10.1111/ina.12751
7. Bowe B, Xie Y, Al-Aly Z. Acute and postacute sequelae associated with SARS-CoV-2 reinfection. Nat Med. 2022;28(11):2398-2405. doi:10.1038/s41591-022-02051-3
8. Shen XR, Geng R, Li Q, et al. ACE2-independent infection of T lymphocytes by SARS-CoV-2. Signal Transduct Target Ther. 2022;7(1):1-11. doi:10.1038/s41392-022-00919-x
9. Li J, Zhou Y, Ma J, et al. The long-term health outcomes, pathophysiological mechanisms and multidisciplinary management of long COVID. Signal Transduct Target Ther. 2023;8(1):1-19. doi:10.1038/s41392-023-01640-z
10. Castanares-Zapatero D, Chalon P, Kohn L, et al. Pathophysiology and mechanism of long COVID: a comprehensive review. Ann Med. 2022;54(1):1473-1487. doi:10.1080/07853890.2022.2076901
11. Bai Y, Tao X. Comparison of COVID-19 and influenza characteristics. J Zhejiang Univ Sci B. 2021;22(2):87-98. doi:10.1631/jzus.B2000479
12. Tracking SARS-CoV-2 variants. Accessed January 20, 2024. https://www.who.int/activities/tracking-SARS-CoV-2-variants
13. Pulliam JRC, van Schalkwyk C, Govender N, et al. Increased risk of SARS-CoV-2 reinfection associated with emergence of Omicron in South Africa. Science. 2022;376(6593):eabn4947. doi:10.1126/science.abn4947
14. Tan ST, Kwan AT, Rodríguez-Barraquer I, et al. Infectiousness of SARS-CoV-2 breakthrough infections and reinfections during the Omicron wave. Nat Med. 2023;29(2):358-365. doi:10.1038/s41591-022-02138-x

15. Davis HE, McCorkell L, Vogel JM, Topol EJ. Long COVID: major findings, mechanisms and recommendations. Nat Rev Microbiol. 2023;21(3):133-146. doi:10.1038/s41579-022-00846-2
16. Gao Z, Xu Y, Sun C, et al. A systematic review of asymptomatic infections with COVID-19. J Microbiol Immunol Infect Wei Mian Yu Gan Ran Za Zhi. 2021;54(1):12-16. doi:10.1016/j.jmii.2020.05.001
17. Rao S, Gross RS, Mohandas S, et al. Postacute Sequelae of SARS-CoV-2 in Children. Pediatrics. Published online February 7, 2024:e2023062570. doi:10.1542/peds.2023-062570
18. Morens DM, Folkers GK, Fauci AS. The Concept of Classical Herd Immunity May Not Apply to COVID-19. J Infect Dis. Published online March 21, 2022:jiac109. doi:10.1093/infdis/jiac109

Chapter 2: The COVID-19 Pandemic and the Media's Role

1. LaPook J. Indoor air systems crucial to curbing spread of viruses, aerosol researchers say - CBS News. Published October 29, 2023. Accessed January 24, 2024. https://www.cbsnews.com/news/indoor-air-quality-healthy-buildings-60-minutes-transcript/
2. Uccello, Cori. Drivers of 2024 Health Insurance Premium Changes. American Academy of Actuaries; 2023. https://www.actuary.org/sites/default/files/2023-07/health-brief-premium-drivers.pdf

Chapter 3: Overview of SARS-CoV-2

1. V'kovski P, Kratzel A, Steiner S, Stalder H, Thiel V. Coronavirus biology and replication: implications for SARS-CoV-2. Nat Rev Microbiol. 2021;19(3):155-170. doi:10.1038/s41579-020-00468-6
2. Bai C, Zhong Q, Gao GF. Overview of SARS-CoV-2 genome-encoded proteins. Sci China Life Sci. 2022;65(2):280-294. doi:10.1007/s11427-021-1964-4
3. Weller SK, Coen DM. Herpes Simplex Viruses: Mechanisms of DNA Replication. Cold Spring Harb Perspect Biol. 2012;4(9):a013011. doi:10.1101/cshperspect.a013011
4. Morens DM, Folkers GK, Fauci AS. The Concept of Classical Herd Immunity May Not Apply to COVID-19. J Infect Dis. Published online March 21, 2022:jiac109. doi:10.1093/infdis/jiac109
5. Ritonavir-Boosted Nirmatrelvir (Paxlovid). COVID-19 Treatment Guidelines. Accessed February 4, 2024.

https://www.covid19treatmentguidelines.nih.gov/therapies/antivirals-including-antibody-products/ritonavir-boosted-nirmatrelvir--paxlovid-/
6. Paxlovid | HHS/ASPR. Accessed February 4, 2024. https://aspr.hhs.gov:443/COVID-19/Therapeutics/Products/Paxlovid/Pages/default.aspx
7. Hammond J, Leister-Tebbe H, Gardner A, et al. Oral Nirmatrelvir for High-Risk, Nonhospitalized Adults with Covid-19. N Engl J Med. 2022;386(15):1397-1408. doi:10.1056/NEJMoa2118542
8. Edelstein GE, Boucau J, Uddin R, et al. SARS-CoV-2 Virologic Rebound With Nirmatrelvir–Ritonavir Therapy. Ann Intern Med. 2023;176(12):1577-1585. doi:10.7326/M23-1756
9. Davis HE, McCorkell L, Vogel JM, Topol EJ. Long COVID: major findings, mechanisms and recommendations. Nat Rev Microbiol. 2023;21(3):133-146. doi:10.1038/s41579-022-00846-2

Chapter 4: Long COVID: More Than Just a Cough

1. Ashraf UM, Abokor AA, Edwards JM, et al. SARS-CoV-2, ACE2 expression, and systemic organ invasion. Physiol Genomics. 2021;53(2):51-60. doi:10.1152/physiolgenomics.00087.2020
2. Davis HE, McCorkell L, Vogel JM, Topol EJ. Long COVID: major findings, mechanisms and recommendations. Nat Rev Microbiol. 2023;21(3):133-146. doi:10.1038/s41579-022-00846-2
3. How many people in the US have long COVID? USAFacts. Accessed January 14, 2024. https://usafacts.org/articles/how-many-people-have-long-covid/
4. Guidance for Certifying Deaths Due to Coronavirus Disease 2019 (COVID–19): Expanded in February 2023 to Include Guidance for Certifying Deaths Due to Post-Acute Sequelae of COVID-19. National Center for Health Statistics (U.S.); 2023. doi:10.15620/cdc:124588
5. Zhouyi Rong, Hongcheng Mai, Saketh Kapoor, et al. SARS-CoV-2 Spike Protein Accumulation in the Skull-Meninges-Brain Axis: Potential Implications for Long-Term Neurological Complications in post-COVID-19. bioRxiv. Published online January 1, 2023:2023.04.04.535604. doi:10.1101/2023.04.04.535604
6. Martínez-Mármol R, Giordano-Santini R, Kaulich E, et al. SARS-CoV-2 infection and viral fusogens cause neuronal and glial fusion that compromises neuronal activity. Sci Adv. 2023;9(23):eadg2248. doi:10.1126/sciadv.adg2248
7. Meng M, Wei R, Wu Y, et al. Long-term risks of respiratory diseases in patients infected with SARS-CoV-2: a longitudinal, population-based cohort study. eClinicalMedicine. 2024;69.

doi:10.1016/j.eclinm.2024.102500
8. Perico L, Benigni A, Casiraghi F, Ng LFP, Renia L, Remuzzi G. Immunity, endothelial injury and complement-induced coagulopathy in COVID-19. Nat Rev Nephrol. 2021;17(1):46-64. doi:10.1038/s41581-020-00357-4
9. Kalaw FGP, Warter A, Cavichini M, et al. Retinal tissue and microvasculature loss in COVID-19 infection. Sci Rep. 2023;13(1):5100. doi:10.1038/s41598-023-31835-x
10. Agbuduwe C, Basu S. Haematological manifestations of COVID-19: From cytopenia to coagulopathy. Eur J Haematol. 2020;105(5):540-546. doi:10.1111/ejh.13491
11. Lymphocytopenia - Hematology and Oncology. Merck Manuals Professional Edition. Accessed August 22, 2023. https://www.merckmanuals.com/professional/hematology-and-oncology/leukopenias/lymphocytopenia
12. Shen XR, Geng R, Li Q, et al. ACE2-independent infection of T lymphocytes by SARS-CoV-2. Signal Transduct Target Ther. 2022;7(1):1-11. doi:10.1038/s41392-022-00919-x
13. Bowe B, Xie Y, Al-Aly Z. Acute and postacute sequelae associated with SARS-CoV-2 reinfection. Nat Med. 2022;28(11):2398-2405. doi:10.1038/s41591-022-02051-3
14. Gonzalez H, Hagerling C, Werb Z. Roles of the immune system in cancer: from tumor initiation to metastatic progression. Genes Dev. 2018;32(19-20):1267-1284. doi:10.1101/gad.314617.118
15. Mallick D, Goyal L, Chourasia P, Zapata MR, Yashi K, Surani S. COVID-19 Induced Postural Orthostatic Tachycardia Syndrome (POTS): A Review. Cureus. 15(3):e36955. doi:10.7759/cureus.36955
16. Haffke M, Freitag H, Rudolf G, et al. Endothelial dysfunction and altered endothelial biomarkers in patients with post-COVID-19 syndrome and chronic fatigue syndrome (ME/CFS). J Transl Med. 2022;20(1):138. doi:10.1186/s12967-022-03346-2
17. Komaroff AL, Lipkin WI. ME/CFS and Long COVID share similar symptoms and biological abnormalities: road map to the literature. Front Med. 2023;10:1187163. doi:10.3389/fmed.2023.1187163
18. Bull-Otterson L. Post–COVID Conditions Among Adult COVID-19 Survivors Aged 18–64 and ≥65 Years — United States, March 2020–November 2021. MMWR Morb Mortal Wkly Rep. 2022;71. doi:10.15585/mmwr.mm7121e1

Chapter 5: Masking: Beyond Individual Choice

1. Dyke MEV. Trends in County-Level COVID-19 Incidence in Counties

With and Without a Mask Mandate — Kansas, June 1–August 23, 2020. MMWR Morb Mortal Wkly Rep. 2020;69. doi:10.15585/mmwr.mm6947e2

2. Lyu W, Wehby GL. Community Use Of Face Masks And COVID-19: Evidence From A Natural Experiment Of State Mandates In The US. Health Aff (Millwood). 2020;39(8):1419-1425. doi:10.1377/hlthaff.2020.00818
3. Howard J, Huang A, Li Z, et al. An evidence review of face masks against COVID-19. Proc Natl Acad Sci U S A. 2021;118(4):e2014564118. doi:10.1073/pnas.2014564118
4. Face Masks and COVID-19. NIH News in Health. Published October 28, 2021. Accessed March 2, 2024. https://newsinhealth.nih.gov/2021/11/face-masks-covid-19
5. Liao M, Liu H, Wang X, et al. A technical review of face mask wearing in preventing respiratory COVID-19 transmission. Curr Opin Colloid Interface Sci. 2021;52:101417. doi:10.1016/j.cocis.2021.101417
6. Luo M, Liu S, Zhu L, et al. Analysis of a super-transmission of SARS-CoV-2 omicron variant BA.5.2 in the outdoor night market. Front Public Health. 2023;11:1153303. doi:10.3389/fpubh.2023.1153303
7. Nwosu ADG, Ossai EN, Onwuasoigwe O, Ahaotu F. Oxygen saturation and perceived discomfort with face mask types, in the era of COVID-19: a hospital-based cross-sectional study. Pan Afr Med J. 2021;39:203. doi:10.11604/pamj.2021.39.203.28266
8. Vishwanath V, Favo CL, Tu TH, et al. Effects of face masks on oxygen saturation at graded exercise intensities. J Osteopath Med. 2023;123(3):167-176. doi:10.1515/jom-2022-0132

Chapter 6: Clean Air

1. Qian H, Zheng X. Ventilation control for airborne transmission of human exhaled bio-aerosols in buildings. J Thorac Dis. 2018;10(Suppl 19):S2295-S2304. doi:10.21037/jtd.2018.01.24
2. Climate Change: Atmospheric Carbon Dioxide | NOAA Climate.gov. Accessed March 9, 2024. http://www.climate.gov/news-features/understanding-climate/climate-change-atmospheric-carbon-dioxide
3. Allen JG, MacNaughton P, Satish U, Santanam S, Vallarino J, Spengler JD. Associations of Cognitive Function Scores with Carbon Dioxide, Ventilation, and Volatile Organic Compound Exposures in Office Workers: A Controlled Exposure Study of Green and Conventional Office Environments. Environ Health Perspect.

2016;124(6):805-812. doi:10.1289/ehp.1510037
4. White LF, Murray EJ, Chakravarty A. The role of schools in driving SARS-CoV-2 transmission: Not just an open-and-shut case. Cell Rep Med. 2022;3(3):100556. doi:10.1016/j.xcrm.2022.100556
5. Rao S, Gross RS, Mohandas S, et al. Postacute Sequelae of SARS-CoV-2 in Children. Pediatrics. Published online February 7, 2024:e2023062570. doi:10.1542/peds.2023-062570
6. Brisbane school avoids COVID outbreak after dads band together, armed with smoke machine. ABC News. https://www.abc.net.au/news/2022-04-01/brisbane-school-no-covid-omicron-outbreaks-term-1/100956850. Published March 31, 2022. Accessed March 10, 2024.
7. LaPook J. Indoor air systems crucial to curbing spread of viruses, aerosol researchers say - CBS News. Published October 29, 2023. Accessed January 24, 2024. https://www.cbsnews.com/news/indoor-air-quality-healthy-buildings-60-minutes-transcript/